FOOD MEDICINE

VOLUME 1

The number 1 Rule for a Long and Healthy Life

DEBORAH HARPER

BALBOA.PRESS

A DIVISION OF HAY HOUSE

Balboa Press books may be ordered through booksellers or by contacting:

Balboa Press
A Division of Hay House
1663 Liberty Drive
Bloomington, IN 47403
www.balboapress.com.au
1 (877) 407-4847

Print information available on the last page.

ISBN: 978-1-5043-2027-6 (sc)
ISBN: 978-1-5043-2028-3 (e)

Balboa Press rev. date: 12/27/2019

DEDICATION

MOTHER

This book is dedicated to all mothers.

We are the traditional nurturers, protectors and the first teachers of our children.

They are the next generation in which we trust the care and nurturing will continue for generation after generation.

Let's examine what have we learnt over the last 50 years and what message we pass on to our children so they can thrive. As long as they are healthy we will have done our job.

When you think about it a generation is merely 25 years.

In 25 years a whole way of life can change.

I found this quote in a book by *Diana Gabaldon:*

Through the Stones.

"You have 4 grandparents, 8 great grandparents, 16 great-great grandparents and 32 great-great-great grandparents. With an average

age of twenty five years between each generation this means that during the past five hundred years, there were 1,048,576 people all contributing to the production of YOU".

That really amazes me, but it also shows how we are all in the same boat. Western European people, like me, for example, suffer from heart disease, cancers, respiratory disease, diabetes and obesity. Many of these diseases are simply lifestyle diseases that can be reversed, or can be avoided altogether. In the next 25 years my hope is we can learn from our mistakes and create a brighter, healthier future for our next generation.

FOREWORD

OUR ARMY OF ALLIES

Picture your body as a car and that you are driving a 2 million year old car.

What fuel do you use?

This car is a natural, organic, living, breathing car.

For 2 million years that car has been using a fuel made up of: water, seeds, nuts, grasses, herbs, roots, fruits, vegetables, grains and meats - after all that is the fuel it is used to.

More importantly that is the kind of fuel it was made for!

Then suddenly after 2 million years on the same fuel that car has to switch over to a new fuel.

In the past 150 years a new and modern mixture has been added to run the car: sugar, sweets, biscuits, crisps, chocolate, cola and soft drinks, processed fats and oils, cigarettes and alcohol, prescription and illegal drugs, chemicals, herbicides, pesticides and preservatives.

What do you think will happen to this 2 million year old natural, organic, living, breathing car?

That's right, it breaks down.

The performance fuel has gone, replaced with a man-made cocktail that the body does not recognize as fuel.

But the body is resilient and adapts. For every new dis-ease that your immune system comes in contact with, cells are alerted, they identify the dis-ease, memorize the dis-ease, and immediately start fighting it.

Your body, providing it is well fuelled, can fight and heal and remember every dis-ease it has come in contact with. You may have a dis-ease right now circulating through your body, but have no symptoms because you've had that dis-ease before and your very intelligent immune system has dealt with it before it has even caused any symptoms.

Such is the wisdom of your body.

Much of the fuel we consume today is polluted and unrecognizable to our bodies.

Now is the time to take note of your allies and avoid your enemies.

I have a saying, **"Fresh is best- forget the rest".** By changing your diet to accommodate the types of foods our bodies recognize as premium fuel you will be rewarded with maximum performance and dependability.

FOOD FOR THOUGHT!

There has been a 37% increase in cancer cases in China since the western diet has replaced the traditional Chinese diet.

"The Greatest Medicine of them all is to teach people how Not to Need it".

And in this book you will learn just how to achieve that goal. It all comes down to following 1 simple rule. Once you know it the rest is easy.

Hi Friend, My name is Debbie Harper,

And I help people create a healthier life and home while saving you money and your environment. I promote "Regenerative Food Medicine" that includes sustainable living practices.

If there was only 1 rule you had to follow for Living a Long and Healthy Life. Would you do it?

If you are suffering from an allergy or illness and you follow this 1 rule you will reduce Your Symptoms and reverse Your Dis-ease altogether.

What if I said if you follow this 1 rule you will Lose Weight Forever and keep it off?

How about if I said by following this 1 rule you could also Save Money.

And if I said by following this 1 rule you could support Local Industry and Local Jobs.

By following this 1 rule you can also Reduce Household Waste.

Follow this 1 rule and you will be helping to Save Your Planet.

And what if I said if you follow this 1 rule you may never have to visit your doctor or never have to worry about medical bills again and provide a better future for our children, Would YOU do it?

ACKNOWLEDGMENTS

1/ Fresh is Best Forget the Rest. "Butters Better"

2/ Fresh Fruit and Vegetables

3/ Supermarkets

4/ Farmers Markets

5/ A Traditional diet

6/ 10 Dangerous Things in the Modern Home

7/ The Whole is Greater than the Sum of its Parts

8/ The 2/3 1/3 Rule

9/ In the Garden

10/Why a healthy diet and saving the planet are the same thing.

BONUS MATERIAL

CHAPTER 1

"FRESH IS BEST FORGET THE REST"

In this first chapter we will look at butter and margarine and compare the difference.

We are just getting started but this example highlights many of the foods we consume today that are doing more harm than good and emphasises just how important it is to **Eat Fresh.**

Let's get started

The 1 rule is:

"Fresh is Best Forget the Rest".

Now that you know the 1 rule you have plenty of time to mull this over as you read this book.

Butters Better.

There was an ad that played on TV here in New Zealand some years ago that showed the difference between butter and margarine

1

quite clearly. It labelled the ingredients of butter, cream and salt and compared it to the ingredients of margarine and the list of ingredients in margarine scrolled on and on. I'll list them now and they will fill this entire page and more……..

The Margarine Story revealed:

Contents:

Vegetable-oil blend

Water

Whey (milk)

Salt

Vegetable mono & diglycerides

Soy lecithin

Citric acid artificial flavours

Vitamin A

Beta carotene (for colour)

And how it is made (which is very disturbing, actually):

Margarine makers start with cheap poor quality vegetable oils, such as corn, cottonseed, soybeans, safflower seeds and canola. These oils have already turned rancid by the way, from being extracted from oil seeds using high temperature (which destroys the oil making it rancid) and high pressure.

Rancid oils are loaded with free radicals that react easily with other molecules, causing cell damage, premature aging and a host of other problems.

The last bit of oil is removed with hexane, a solvent known to cause cancer. Although this hexane is later removed, traces of it are unavoidably left behind.

Unfit for human consumption

Moreover, some of these oils are not suitable for human consumption to begin with. Cottonseed oil, one of the most popular margarine ingredients, has natural toxins and unrefined cottonseed oil is used as a pesticide. The toxin, gossypol, is removed during refining though.

Cottonseed oil also contains far too much Omega-6 fatty acids in relation to Omega 3.

While both Omega 6 and Omega 3 are essential fatty acids, an imbalance between the two is widely believed to cause various health problems, including heart disease.

Most experts on the subject believe that a healthy ratio of omega 3 to omega 6 is between 1:1 and 1:2. Cotton seed oil, however, has over 50 percent omega 6 and only trace amounts of Omega 3, giving a ratio of 1: several hundred or more.

Cotton is also one of the most heavily sprayed crops, there are concerns that cottonseed oil may be highly contaminated with pesticide residues. However, insufficient testing has been done to provide proof.

Canola oil, is widely touted as the healthiest oil of all. But canola oil has problems as well.

Consumption of Canola has been linked with vitamin E deficiency as well as growth retardation.

For this reason, Canola oil is not allowed to be used in the manufacture of infant formula.

The oils used for making margarine are also among the Big Four genetically modified crops – soy, corn, rapeseed / Canola and cotton.

The raw oils for making margarine are steam cleaned. This destroys all the vitamins and antioxidants. However, the residues of pesticides and solvents – that is, hexane – remain.

The oils are mixed with finely ground nickel, a highly toxic substance that serves as a catalyst for the chemical reaction during the hydrogenation process.

Other catalysts may be used, but these, too, are highly toxic. The oils are then put under high temperature and pressure in a reactor. Hydrogen gas is introduced. The high temperature and pressure, together with the presence of the nickel catalyst, causes hydrogen atoms to be forced into the oil molecules.

This helps to make it solid.

No longer polyunsaturated fat

From this processing trans-fats are formed during partial hydrogenation. These are fat molecules that have been twisted out of shape. In liquid oils, the molecules are bent, with the hydrogen atoms on opposite sides of each other.

During partial hydrogenation, the molecules are somewhat straightened and now all the hydrogen molecules are on the same side. If the oil is fully hydrogenated, it turns into a hard solid that cannot be eaten.

It no longer contains trans-fats because the "out of shape" oil molecules have all been broken up to form straight chains. But this does not mean they have become healthy again because of all the unnatural steps above.

What comes out of the partial hydrogenation process is a smelly, lumpy, grey grease.

To remove the lumps, emulsifiers – which are like soaps – are mixed in. The oil is steam cleaned (again!) to remove the odour of chemicals.

This step is called deodorization and it again involves high temperature and high pressure.

The oil is then bleached to get rid of the grey colour.

Synthetic vitamins and artificial flavours are mixed in.

A natural yellow colour is added to margarine, as synthetic colouring is not allowed!

(Wow! After the horse has bolted).

In fact, early last century, all colouring was not allowed and margarine was white.

This was to protect consumers so that they did not get butter and margarine mixed up.

Finally, the margarine is promoted to the public as a health food – with the full endorsement of many scientists, doctors, nutritionists and health authorities.

Wow that was quite a few processes! This ad was very simple but effective. Because it showed how pure and easy butter is to make compared to margarine and the margarine story is not a good one.

"Where margarine is consumed in significant quantities, the rate of heart attack is higher"

<u>10 Healthy Reasons to enjoy Real Butter</u>

Oh!

And by the way **butter is better** and you can make your own. I'd like to see you try and make margarine! Take some cream with a pinch of salt put in a container with a lid on tight and shake.

That's it, shake it.

Now it's solid – after all that shaking, squeeze the butter, remove the butter milk (which is the remaining liquid) and feed it to baby!

Yeah that's right, the butter milk from making butter is not wasted, it is dried and reused in infant formula.

Safe for baby and pretty simple eh!

Back to margarine: Margarine and any similar vegetable fat is not the health benefit we are lead to believe it is.

While it is advertised as polyunsaturated fat, it is not really true. Manufacturers neglect to mention the process of making margarine and any similar vegetable fat **solid**, creates a "new artificially hydrogenated vegetable fat" which is essentially synthetic food that the human body has no experience with.

The reason I have used the margarine story first up in this book is to highlight what we have done with the food we consume today.

The question is: *"Is it the food I'm eating that is bad for me or is it what they have done to the food I am eating that is bad for me"*. <u>Robyn O'Brien</u> *(The Erin Brockovich of food)*.

Margarine is just one example there are many more. My area of expertise is with nutrition. I acknowledge mental and physical wellbeing are just as important to living a healthy life but I do not feel qualified to talk about them. My only contribution to physical wellbeing is walking. I try to get in a 30 minute walk daily in the fresh air, I enjoy gardening too. Whatever you do for exercise it must be a joy to you not a chore. For mental wellbeing I would have to say "be happy" treasure all the joyful, happy, enthusiastic moments in your life and be at peace. Face the hard times with courage and recognition. Do not dwell on the negative. See beauty in all things and you will live a more vibrant life.

CHAPTER 2

In chapter two we look at common foods that are our allies in health. These foods have been used for centuries as medicines. We also compare foods that are commonly eaten today with their healthier equivalent and investigate some foods considered 'good for you' that could be responsible for illness, allergies and weight gain.

Fresh fruit and fresh vegetables.

Always choose fresh fruit and vegetables where possible. Home grown fruit and vegetables are the best. Next best would have to be the farmers markets.

When you taste an apple straight from the tree something wonderful happens. Your taste buds are rewarded with the crisp crack and crunch, the awesome juiciness of the fresh white flesh and the flavour of freshness. This out performs anything you can buy at the supermarket. Because try as they may they just can't deliver anything to you that is that as fresh especially when they are out of season. The only time is when the apple is in season and from your own country.

So, how long do apples last?

When properly stored, the shelf life of fresh apples past their sell by date is approximately: 2-4 weeks in the pantry or 1-2 months refrigerated.

Ever bitten into an apple from the supermarket and found it was rotten floury or bruised inside? Grrrrr!

Fruit Juices

Say no to any fruit juice as well, if you don't want huge amounts of fructose sugar in your diet. Removing the fibre turns fruit juice into a sugary drink as harmful as coke.

The fruit juices you find at the supermarket aren't always what they seem. They may have small amounts of real fruit in them, but often they are little more than water, artificial flavour, added vitamin's and sugar. Orange juice is a very good example because for as many varieties on the market there are just as many differing levels of ingredients.

But even if you're drinking real fruit juice, that you have made yourself from fresh, it is **still a bad idea to have too much.** Fruit juice is like fruit with most of the good stuff removed. All that is left is the sugar and a few vitamins. There's no fibre in it, no chewing resistance and nothing to stop you from downing massive amounts of sugar in a short amount of time. Eating too much sugar is associated with all sorts of diseases including obesity, type II diabetes, cardiovascular disease and many others. It is much better for you to avoid fruit juices and eat real whole fruits from the tree instead.

For example the humble apple.

THE HUMBLE APPLE TREE

Remember the saying, "An apple a day keeps the doctor away"?

"If you could plant only one tree in your garden it should be an apple."

Says famous French Herbalist Maurice Messegue. (1)

From an apple tree you can eat the fruit fresh, preserve by drying or boiling, and make sauce as well as apple cider vinegar which is reputed to be one of the world's first medicines.

An apple tree is a must.

If you have enough room plant an early, a medium and a late fruiting variety for a longer season. You can plant your fruit trees on the border of your section as close as 2 metres apart; the branches will tangle into each other which has the advantage of keeping the birds away even if you need a ladder to reach the fruit.

Another way is to train your apple tree on to a trellis which will flatten out the branches (espalier) - in this way your fruit tree can double as a good border fence; or up against a north facing wall of your shed or retaining wall.

Take advantage of any north facing (if you're in the southern hemisphere) area in your garden to maximize the most of the sunlight; also consider terracing, placing lower growing plants to the front and progressively taller plants at the rear if space is an issue.

More on Apples

Apple cider vinegar can be used in your house hold cleaning especially if infused with a bunch of aromatic antibacterial germ killing herbs such as Lavender, Mint, Thyme, and Rosemary.

Apple cider vinegar is an old folk remedy claimed to be beneficial in treating a long list of ailments. A great detoxifier, for those suffering from arthritis, rheumatism or gout. A guard against osteoporosis, acid reflux, heartburn and gas formation:

Lowers blood pressure and cholesterol,

Thins thickened blood,

Prevents cancer,

Destroys infection,

Relieves night time cramps,

Soothes sprained muscles,

Eases headaches,

Relieves corns,

Relieves callas,

Athlete's foot,

Insect bites and sunburn,

A remedy for urinary tract infections,

Destroys bacteria in food,

Detoxifies fruit and vegetable sprays,

Assists in digestion and weight control,

Maintains memory and protects the mind from aging.

Amazing ☺

AC Vinegar is said to have been used for 10,000 years. The Babylonians first converted wine into vinegar in 5000 BC using date palms, grapes and figs believing in its exceptional healing properties.

Hippocrates (considered the founder of medicine) used vinegar as an antibiotic. Samurai warriors used vinegar as a tonic for strength and power. During the US Civil War, soldiers used vinegar to prevent gastric upset and as a treatment for various ailments including pneumonia and scurvy. It was used to treat wounds during World War 1.

Modern medical research identifies beta-carotene in apple cider vinegar as destroying free radicals in the body. Free radicals are involved in the aging and mutation of tissues and in destroying the immune system.

Apple cider vinegar's beta-carotene is said to be in a 'natural, easy to digest form'. The pectin found in apples works through the digestive system binding to cholesterol and removing it from the body. US studies (2) have shown pectin (3) also protects us from the ravages of pollution, binding to heavy metals such as lead or mercury in the body and carrying them safely out.

Malic and tartaric acids in apples help neutralize the acid by products of digestion, and help your body to cope with excess protein or rich fatty food.

In a fascinating series of tests described by Jean Carper in, *"The Food Pharmacy"*, virologist Dr Jack Konowalchuk and colleague Joan Speirs from Canada's Bureau of <u>Microbial Hazards (4)</u> exposed a wide range of viruses in tissue cell cultures to a number of fruit juices including blueberry, cranberry, grape, plum, pomegranate, raspberry, strawberry and apple juice, taken off a supermarket shelf.

After 24 hours almost none of the viruses survived. The researchers remained unsure just what substance in the apple – pulp or juice or skin had had this effect - certainly they're present even in commercial juice. Probably one of our biggest health concerns with many people today is acid reflux and heartburn from pour digestion. If left to escalate this will only cause more health problems.

The most useful reason for drinking ACV daily is its ability to neutralise an over acid stomach. Many people suffer from acid reflux and heartburn and seek relief from prescription drugs.

<u>Losec</u> (5) is one of these drugs and I find the method of action is debatable. Drugs such as Losec reduce or stop hydrochloric acid production which in turn eliminates the symptoms.

But hydrochloric acid breaks down food and more importantly absorbs nutrients and transports them through the body. And to reduce or stop hydrochloric acid production seems erroneous.

Many moons ago. My brother and I were on holiday. Just doing a bit of shopping, he had a prescription to pick up for Losec. Naturally because of my background in natural health I was concerned that he was taking it but hey this is my big brother.

We're on holiday. I'm not about to preach to him. So I mentioned that I thought probiotics could be very helpful too.

He had to get his prescription filled and we were in a mall in Dunedin. I spotted the chemist and we headed for this escalator. As we come up the escalator I was blown away to see in neon lights "and Herbal Dispensary" alongside the chemists sign.

People who live in Dunedin will remember this chemist. Anyway we went in and I headed for the probiotics and my brother headed for the counter to get his prescription filled.

As I got to the counter I heard the chemist saying, "Oh god no that stuff ill kill yah!" I couldn't believe it the chemist was telling my brother that <u>Losec (5)</u> was not going to help him long term.

I put the probiotics down on the counter and said "will this help" and the chemist said yes, and carried on talking to my brother.

I was rapt.

This guy was giving my brother excellent advice and strategies to reduce his need for medication. Naturally I wanted to tell my brother about those things, but I didn't feel it would make any impact on him.

But the chemist on the other hand couldn't have helped him more by telling him he has an active role in his wellness and here are some of the tools.

Getting back to lovely fresh apples I can vouch for ACV to assist in reducing acid reflux almost immediately because it causes your pH levels to become more alkaline. Acidic pH balance will discourage bacteria, yeast and fungal growth and prevent poisons from reaching the systems of the body.

ACV will also improve the health of dairy cows, horses, dogs and other animals by reducing

common infections; ACV is an aid in whelping, improves stamina, prevents muscle fatigue after exercise, increases resistance to disease, reduces intestinal and faecal odours and protects against food poisoning.

You may feel inclined to make your very own ACV. And there are plenty of recipes on the internet. I strongly suggest you google 'Organic apple cider vinegar'. Although some sights may urge you to boil your vinegar nothing will be as beneficial as the raw food with the live mother included. The mother is the jelly-like sediment, which can be saved and used in the next batch to get everything started.

Organic apple cider vinegar is a fantastic base to make your own household cleaning agents too. Its antiseptic qualities make it the perfect partner to some antiseptic, antibacterial herbs.

As well as preserving beneficial herbs to use in cleaning, you can also choose culinary herbs for cooking and aromatic herbs for cosmetics.

They would be the only cosmetics, food and cleaning product that you could clean your face and floors and eat.

Sounds pretty safe to me!

If you're not yet completely convinced about the benefits of vinegar.

Check out this little bit of history.

We have all heard about the Black Plague, known as the Black Death killing an estimated one third the population in the first major outbreak around 1346 – 1453 with more sporadic outbreaks for 400 hundred years.

Today we have learnt from DNA analysis that the pathogen responsible was most likely Yersinia-Pestis bacterium. And while most people were running around blaming this pestilence on Sin and a punishment from god. Somebody had to comfort the sick and handle the dead. The ingenious solution was fortification with herbs and vinegar.

Physicians clothed themselves in long robes, wide brimmed hats and donned masks with long beaks. These beaks held dried herbs, spices and essential oils which the physician breathed. The robe and hat were also doused in this brew. And from this brew came the well-known remedy called <u>"four thieves vinegar" (6)</u>

Named for some enterprising thieves who would enter the homes of the dying or dead and rob them blind.

At the time this astonished the authorities, they could not believe anyone would be so foolish as to risk death and enter the homes of the dying.

But it also worked extremely well. Scientific evidence today proves that many of these harmful microbes could not live when exposed to these herbs. Imagine then being able to use this preparation to clean your home.

Or as an effective Antibacterial?

There has been plenty of news lately telling us that antibiotics are failing us now because of their overuse. Maybe Four Thief's Vinegar and the like be the solution?

Four Thieves Vinegar.

Marseilles Vinegar. – For Thieves' Vinegar.

Prophylactic Vinegar. Vinaigre des Quatre

Voleurs, Acetum Quator Furum. The original

Formula for this once celebrated preparation

Is: Rosemary tops, dried .... 4 oz.

Sage flowers, dried .... 4 oz.

Lavender flowers, dried............. 2 oz.

Rue, fresh ....1 ½ oz.

Camphor, dissolved in spirit...... .1 oz.

Garlic, sliced........................ ¼ oz.

Cloves, bruised .... 1 drm.

Distilled wine vinegar, strongest 1 gal.

Digest for 7 or 8 days with occasional agitation, pour off the liquor, press out the remainder, and filter the mixed liquids.

It is said that this medicated vinegar was invented by four thieves of Marseilles, who successfully employed it, as a prophylactic, during a visitation of pestilence.

Making Tinctures

Let's make some tinctures, which is a way of extracting beneficial constituents from selected herbs.

How to make a tincture for home use

First dry the herbs you need. This can be done in by collecting the plant material on a dry sunny day after the dew is dried off. Mint, Garlic, Rosemary. Sage. Lavender, Thyme are all great additions for this brew. Bundle together in small bunches and hang to dry.

If you have a hot water cupboard this is best but just hanging in the kitchen will be fine.

Plant material is dry when they crunch when squeezed.

In 2-3 weeks most herbs are dry using this method.

Chop the freshly dried herb and pack into a clean, sterilized jar and pour over ACV to cover herb.

Seal jar with a plastic lid and place in a dark place for 2 – 6 weeks. Check and shake jar daily to ensure herb material is well covered by ACV.

Remove plant material and discard onto your compost heap.

Place remaining infused ACV into a sterilized bottle with a non-metal lid, and label

All preparations should have the following information on your label:

Name of plant material used

Type of preparation process

Date of preparation and date of bottling as well as the expiry date

Vinegar tinctures made this way will keep up to 2 years. Do not use the boiling vinegar, use only organic apple cider vinegar from your health food store or local apple growers. Do not use metal caps as these will corrode. Vinegars can be used as a medicinal preparation or in cooking, cleaning and salads.

As mention earlier in this book some of the best herbs for all of the above uses are: Mint, Lavender, Thyme, Rosemary and also Sage as well as the king of the herbs Garlic.

Tip: Sage infused in water makes a great deodorant for personal use.

Gargle with sage if you have a saw throat, add some local honey to soothe and relieve.

Sage will also reduce those hot flushes girls!

Pour 3 cups of boiling water over a handful of fresh or dried herb and infuse for 20 minutes.

Drink 1 cup three times daily until symptoms settle.

Check out "the king of the herbs" here in more detail because it is such an important food medicine.

GARLIC - King of the Herbs

FAMILY: LILIACEAE

Garlic has 4000 years of human history and has been both cherished and reviled. Sought after for its healing powers and shunned for its pungent after effects. From miracle drug to vampire repellent, to offerings for the gods, this unassuming plant has had a prominent place in human history for millennia. And today enjoys a renewed surge in popularity as modern medicine and ancient super food. The bulbs, when roasted are sweet and make a delicious spread. The fresh green tops can be cut for salads and soups giving a strong garlic flavour.

Garlic is grown all over the world originating in Asia for use in food and medicine.

PROPAGATION

As the saying goes - plant on the shortest day, harvest on the longest. The cloves are usually planted in mid-winter because garlic requires a period of chilling below 10°C before hours of long day light and the hot dry conditions of spring and summer.

However garlic can be grown as a perennial herb as long as it is sheltered from the worst frosts. You should be able to grow it all year round - just keep a supply in the ground at all times. Harvest when the tops begin to yellow. Plait them together and hang in your kitchen to dry off and use.

PROPERTIES:

Garlic is anti-septic, anti-viral, anti-microbial and an insecticide. This means it is a valuable aid to healthy pest resistant plants in the garden, as well as an aid to wellness in the body. Use on all fruit trees and bushes, all vegetables in the garden, your valued roses and in the body.

Garlic taken raw internally also helps reduce blood pressure by thinning the blood and cleansing the blood of fatty deposits and microscopic organisms. The volatile oil in garlic is also an expectorant to the lungs clearing mucus and inflammation. The allicin in raw crushed garlic has been shown to kill 23 types of bacteria, including salmonella and staphylococcus.

Heated garlic gives off another compound, <u>diallyl disulphide-oxide</u> <u>(7)</u>, which has been shown to lower serum cholesterol by preventing clotting in the arteries.

Vitamins in garlic, such as A, B, and C, stimulate the body to fight carcinogens and get rid of toxins, and may even aid in preventing certain types of cancer, such as stomach cancer.

Garlic's sulphur compounds can regulate blood sugar metabolism, stimulate and detoxify the liver, and stimulate the blood circulation and the nervous system.

GARLIC in ANTIQUITY

Garlic has been employed in a variety of functions for millennia. Archaeologists have discovered clay sculptures of garlic bulbs and paintings of garlic dating about 3200 B.C. in Egyptian tombs.

A recently discovered Egyptian papyrus dating from 1,500 B.C. recommends garlic as a cure-all for over 22 common ailments, including lack of stamina, heart disease and tumours.

It's also been said the Egyptians fed garlic to the slaves building the pyramids to increase their strength.

Garlic proved itself worthy to peasant and royalty alike as Tutankhamen (Egypt's youngest pharaoh) was sent into the afterlife with garlic at his side.

In ancient Greece and Rome, garlic enjoyed a variety of uses, from repelling scorpions to treating dog bites and bladder infections, to curing leprosy and asthma.

It was even given up as an offering to the Greek goddess Hectate who was the goddess of magic, witchcraft, the night, moon, ghosts and necromancy.

Early Greek military leaders fed garlic to their troops before battles to give them courage and promise victory (and perhaps in an attempt to fell the opposing army with one good whiff.)

Even Greek Olympic athletes counted on garlic to stimulate performance.

In the Middle Ages garlic was thought to combat the plague and was hung in braided strands across the entrances of houses to prevent evil spirits from entering.

Today we would call that "evil spirit" a virus do you think?

For many years, garlic was shunned by Western cultures such as Britain and America because of the residual stench it left behind. In seventeenth century England, garlic was considered unfit for ladies and anyone who wished to court them, and it was avoided even into the 20th century, when famous Chefs would substitute onion for it in recipes.

Beyond superstition, modern research has confirmed what our ancestors already knew about the health benefits of garlic.

In 1858, Louis Pasteur documented that garlic kills bacteria (8), with one millilitre of raw garlic juice proving as effective as 60 milligrams of penicillin.

During World War II, when penicillin and sulphur drugs were scarce, the British and Russian armies used diluted garlic solutions as an antiseptic to disinfect open wounds and prevent gangrene. Though not completely understood at the time, today's research has confirmed that garlic's healing powers stem from hundreds of volatile sulphur compounds found in the vegetable, including allicin, (which gives garlic its offensive odour), alliin, cycroalliin, and diallyl disulphide.

In many cultures garlic is also considered a powerful aphrodisiac and a vegetarian alternative to Viagra. (Wow, only to someone with no sense of smell!)

In Palestinian tradition, a groom who wears a clove of garlic in his buttonhole is guaranteed a happy wedding night.

Some say it's even able to raise a man's sperm count.

Apparently in recent years the kiwi male's sperm count has halved in two decades from about 110 million to 50 million. But good news – boys it is still above the normal level of more than 20 million.

While experts vary in opinion regarding the recommended daily amount of dietary garlic, most of them agree that fresh garlic is better than supplements. To negate the aromatic after effects of fresh garlic, herbalists recommend munching on fresh parsley (it's more than just a garnish, folks) or fennel seed. After about a week of using garlic daily the body should be used to it, and absorb the smell of garlic on the skin.

Garlic supplements abound and people are clamouring for more of the bulbous herb, which complements other recently recognized 'superfoods', such as olive oil and tomato sauce.

Although sometimes maligned, garlic has had an amazing array of nutritional and medicinal applications throughout human history.

And it is still improving the health of the people who use it today.

So grab a clove and enjoy the many benefits of Nature's Oldest Superfood!

Garlic is a Wonderful General Tonic.

In Russia garlic has been traditionally used to keep old age at bay.

Daily use aids and supports the body in a way no other herb does.

Garlic promotes cellular uptake of oxygen and helps circulate it to every cell in your body.

Onions share many of the therapeutic powers of garlic but to a lesser extent.

Garlic is a most effective anti-microbial herb providing zinc, chromium and other nutrients that kill off microbes. Also acting on bacteria, viruses and alimentary parasites. As in *"four thieves vinegar"*. The volatile oil is an effective agent and is largely excreted via the lungs. It is used for bronchitis, respiratory catarrh, recurrent colds and influenza.

As part of a broader approach, garlic is useful in whooping cough and asthma. Garlic will support natural bacteria flora in the gut while killing pathogenic organisms; use for colic, flatulence, food poisoning, worm infestation and dysentery.

Garlic will reduce high blood pressure and normalize cholesterol levels.

An Indian study found that the risk of a second heart attack was greatly reduced by eating four fresh cloves of garlic a day. I would suggest anybody considering taking garlic as a therapeutic aid especially to protect the heart from long term stress would benefit from adding garlic to their daily diet.

For immune enhancing benefits garlic works best by soaking a garlic clove in oil and swallowing whole followed by a large glass of water.

Cooked garlic and garlic capsules benefit the heart but have fewer immune protecting benefits.

If you rub a fresh clove of garlic on the heel of your foot you can soon smell it on your breath - indication enough for me that garlic is all powerful.

In the kitchen use garlic in dressings, butters, vegetarian, meat, egg and all savoury dishes.

ROASTED GARLIC

Place whole garlic bulbs in roasting dish and moderately sprinkle with olive oil. Cook in a moderate oven (180 degrees) for 20 minutes.

Scoop out flesh and eat with breads, crackers and cheese etc.

Roasted garlic is remarkably sweet and a lovely complement to dressings and vegetable dishes. Try roasted garlic aioli dressing for a nice change.

AIOLI

12 cloves of roasted garlic cooled.

3 egg yolks,

1 ¾ cups olive oil,

Salt and pepper to flavour and a few drops of lemon juice.

In your electric blender, first blend garlic slowly adding egg yolks one at a time. Then drizzle in the oil and lemon juice slowly to allow a nice creamy mixture.

When well blended add salt and pepper to taste if required.

You need never buy mayo again.

This recipe is a fraction of the cost of buying ready-made.

GARLIC OIL

Mince fresh garlic cloves into a sterilized jar and cover with oil, carefully removing all air bubbles, and steep for ten days to six weeks.

Use for cooking.

And at the first sign of a cold mix ½ tsp of garlic in oil to 2 tsp organic Manuka honey and the juice of one lemon.

Add this to 250mls of hot water and drink while hot, 3-6 times that day.

GARLIC SYRUP

In a suitable sterile glass jar pour 500gms of peeled and minced garlic and cover with 50/50 apple cider vinegar and water. Cover with a plastic (non-metal) lid and stand for 4 days in a place where you will remember to shake it several times. Add 1 cup of glycerine and stand another day.

Strain and squeeze through a muslin cloth.

Add 1 cup of honey, shake well and store in the fridge.

Use in cooking and as a daily tonic. 1 tsp a day.

Also use as a daily face wash for teenagers suffering from acne.

Dilute the above recipe in 50/50 mix of the syrup and warm water.

Also helpful is to squeeze the juice of a fresh garlic clove directly onto a pimple to help it mature.

Can sting a little though.

MUCUS REDUCING FORMULA

For winter colds, flu and allergens that create copious mucus take one medium onion diced thinly, one inch square piece of fresh ginger diced thinly and a bulb of garlic crushed.

Place in a sterilized jar and pour over honey to cover. (Cold pressed Manuka honey best).

Leave overnight.

Next day strain and discard plant material on your compost heap, reserve liquid and store in an air tight jar in fridge. **Take 1-6tsp daily.**

As a preventative for winter colds 1tsp per day is sufficient.

Take up to 6tsp per day in the acute stage of any infection. Use ½ the adult dose for children.

ONIONS

Onions have been cultivated for more than 5000 years.

Research shows that onions were probably consumed by pre historic man although they may not have cultivated them they grew wild in many parts of the world.

While the place and time of the onion's origin are still a mystery, there are many documents, from very early times, which describe its importance as a food and its use in art, medicine and mummification.

In the time of the Pharaohs, the Egyptians worshipped onions as a symbol of eternity because it was believed the scent was so strong it could wake the dead.

Onions were commonly used in mummification often found in the pelvic regions of the body, in the thorax, flattened against the ears, in front of the collapsed eyes, attached to the soles of the feet and along the legs. Flowering onions have been found on the chest.

King Ramses IV, who died in 1160 B.C., was entombed with onions in his eye sockets.

The Egyptians saw eternal life in the anatomy of the onion because of its circle-within-a-circle structure.

Paintings of onions appear on the inner walls of the pyramids and in the tombs of both the Old Kingdom and the New Kingdom.

The onion is mentioned as a funeral offering and onions are depicted on the banquet tables of the great feasts - both large, peeled onions and slender, immature ones. They were shown upon the altars of the gods.

Frequently, a priest is pictured holding onions in his hand or covering an altar with a bundle of their leaves or roots.

Throughout history the onion has been revered and used in medicine. Known to be a diuretic, good for digestion, the heart, the eyes and the joints.

Greek athletes would consume onions before competing in the Olympic Games, drinking onion juice and rubbing onions on their bodies.

Roman soldiers famous for walking massive distances ate onions regularly and carried them on their journeys to distant lands.

Pliny the Elder, catalogued the Roman beliefs about the efficacy of the onion to cure vision, induce sleep and heal mouth sores, dog bites, toothaches, dysentery and lumbago.

Onions were so prized they were also used as rent payments and wedding gifts.

American Indians used wild onions in syrups, as poultices, as an ingredient in dyes and even as toys.

According to diaries of American colonists, bulb onions were planted as soon as the Pilgrim Fathers could clear the land in 1648.

Onions may be one of the earliest cultivated crops because they were less perishable than other foods of the time, they were transportable, easy to grow and could be grown in a variety of soils and climates. In addition, the onion was useful for sustaining human life.

Onions prevented thirst and could be dried and preserved for later consumption when food might be scarce.

GROWING

Onions prefer a sunny position with a rich but light soil – however they will do well in most soils as long as it is firm. For this reason it is best to prepare the soil well in advance of planting.

Dig the soil to 45cm (18in) deep, working in any organic matter available –remove any stones in the soil during the digging.

Just before planting, tread the soil down so that it is firm. Onions are ideal plants for growing in small confined spaces and they particularly thrive in raised beds.

Today we eat onions as part of our daily diet - some people enjoy them raw. They are included in salads, stews, soups, pickles and accompany many dishes.

Medicinal Uses:

Onions belong to the same botanical family as Garlic and share common compounds the most important being sulphur and quercetin strong antioxidants known to neutralize free radical damage in the body and protect the membrane of cells.

Sulphur is called the "beauty mineral" because it keeps your hair glossy and smooth and keeps the complexion clear and youthful, essential to man, it makes up to 0.25% of human body weight.

There is more sulphur than salt in the body with the highest concentrations found in the joints, hair, skin and nails. Sulphur also has an important relationship with protein, necessary for collagen synthesis, found in insulin a hormone that regulates CHO metabolism, plays a part in tissue respiration, works with the liver to secrete bile and helps maintain overall body balance.

<u>Sulphur</u>(9) is also known as the great cleanser.

Quercetin specifically helps reduce mucus that builds up in the sinuses, an important bioflavonoid in immune support. These compounds help with many common ailments, consuming one raw onion daily, can raise blood levels of good cholesterol by as much as 30%.

They have a useful range of medicinal benefits, among them anaemia, bronchitis and asthma, urinary infections, arthritis and rheumatism, gout and premature aging.

They star in hundreds of traditional recipes.

Colic for babies: Slice an onion, infuse in hot water, cool and give the baby a teaspoon of the water. Many of the historical medicinal uses for onions are now being confirmed in modern research.

Onions have even been shown to be more effective than <u>insulin</u> to lower blood sugar levels in studies with rabbits, subcutaneous injections of onion extract lowered blood sugar levels more slowly than insulin, but for a longer period. It is thought this action is due to the glucokinin in onions.

They are also strongly diuretic, dissolving and eliminating urea, and they have powerful antibiotic activity. One of my favourite ways of using onions is Curry sauce - I have a recipe that my grandmother used which I use as frequently as I can in winter to ward off winter ills and chills.

CURRY SAUCE

4 medium onions,

50 grams butter,

1 tablespoon of hot curry powder or paste,

250ml chicken stock,

Dessert spoon of your favourite chutney.

Peel and chop onions.

Melt the butter in a deep frying pan and add the onion. Cook on a low heat until they are brown (caramelized), stir occasionally to make sure they don't stick to the bottom of the pan.

Take off the heat, cool and mix in all other ingredients, then puree. The quantity of curry powder or paste can be altered to your tastes.

This is a great hearty sauce that can accompany any meat or vegetarian dish.

Fresh Meat and Fish.

A pork roast is better than ham or bacon. Roast beef is better than silverside or corned beef. The process to make ham, bacon and corned beef all add huge amounts of salt. Sausages are the same just another process that devalues the quality of meat.

Shop wisely, not all sausages are mass made. Some boutique outlets make a health conscious gourmet handmade sausage that is perfectly acceptable. This also applies to any meat you buy. Find the best sources for your meat.

If you are lucky enough to have friends or family on a farm I recommend home kill at least you know where it came from and how it lived its life and was packed!

Especially pork as the publicity uncovered by some animal activists on the conditions pigs live in before they arrive on your plate would put you off wanting to eat pork ever again.

Have you seen the pictures of rats running over the pigs who are crowded into pens sometimes alongside other dead pigs!

Avoid any processed meat where possible. This includes any packaged meat product, crumbed product or pre-packaged meals.

UPDATED – 5/22/2013 –

The World Cancer Research Fund (WCRF) has completed a detailed review of more than 7,000 clinical studies covering links between diet and cancer (10).

Bottom line:

Processed meats are too dangerous for human consumption. Consumers should stop buying and eating all processed meat products *for the rest of their lives.*

Processed meats include bacon, sausage, hot dogs, sandwich meat, packaged ham, pepperoni, salami and virtually all red meat used in frozen prepared meals. They are usually manufactured with a carcinogenic ingredient known as sodium nitrite. This is used as a colour fixer by meat companies to turn packaged meats a bright red colour so they look fresh. Unfortunately, sodium nitrite also results in the formation of cancer-causing nitrosamines in the human body. And this leads to a sharp increase in cancer risk for those who eat them.

A 2005 University of Hawaii study found that processed meats increase the risk of pancreatic cancer by <u>67 percent (11)</u>.

Another study revealed that every 50 grams of processed meat consumed daily increases the risk of colorectal cancer by 21 percent.

These are alarming numbers! Note that these cancer risks do not come from eating fresh, non-processed meats. They only appear in people who regularly consume processed meat products containing sodium nitrite. Sodium nitrite appears predominantly in red meat products (you won't find it in chicken or fish products).

Here's a short list of food items to check carefully for sodium nitrite and monosodium glutamate (MSG), another dangerous additive:

Beef jerky

Bacon

Sausage

Sandwich meat

Hot dogs

Frozen pizza with meat

Canned soups with meat

Frozen meals with meat

Ravioli and meat pasta foods

Kid's meals containing red meat

Sandwich meat used at popular restaurants

If <u>sodium nitrite is so dangerous</u> (12) to humans, why do the FDA and USDA continue to allow this cancer-causing chemical to be used? The answer, of course, is that food industry interests now dominate the actions by government regulators.

The USDA, for example, tried to ban sodium nitrite in the late 1970's but was overridden by the meat industry. It insisted the chemical was safe and accused the <u>USDA of trying to "ban bacon."(13)</u>

Consumers are offered no real protection from dangerous chemicals intentionally added to foods, medicines and personal care products. You can protect yourself and your family from the dangers of processed meats by following a few simple rules:

Always read Ingredient labels.

Don't buy anything made with sodium nitrite or monosodium glutamate.

And finally eat only fresh produce with every meal.

There is evidence that natural vitamin C found in citrus fruits and exotic berries help prevent the formation of cancer-causing nitrosamines, protecting you from the devastating health effects of sodium nitrite in processed meats.

The best defence of course, is to avoid eating processed meats altogether. To manage your health and to reduce weight all you have to do is only eat fresh.

The historical use of pork and apple, chicken and herbs stuffing (sage, rosemary and thyme) and beef and rosemary all have one thing in common, the addition of bacteria killing herbs. We have covered the benefits of apples above and when you look at the history it seems that the combination of apples and pork is merely a healthy accident. In traditional times pigs were commonly finished in apple orchards where they ate the apples that had fallen to the ground. This was also around the time the animal would be killed for eating. Another benefit from this practice was that the meat being quite acid was rendered more palatable and the apple helped with digesting the fat.

Chicken and the use of stuffing with known germ killing herbs such as sage, rosemary and thyme would have successfully reduced the risk of bacteria forming. The addition of garlic, thyme and cloves would protect against salmonella poisoning too.

Lamb and rosemary, also have an interesting history. Rosemary is a muscle relaxant as well as an antioxidant. Lamb is a tougher meat and goes well with the flavour of rosemary that just happens to relax the meat when cooked.

Grains

Always choose Organic Whole Grains.

For most people positively the very best start to the day is organic whole grain oats. Porridge is legendary in Scotland, responsible for keeping the average Scottish farmer alive in a harsh climate and commonly all the food they had to survive.

OATS

FAMILY: POACEAE

Avena sativa

I love porridge and have it for breakfast daily all year round. I have been known to take it on holiday with me and have it for lunch if I missed out at breakfast.

Crazy eh! ☺

I love the flavour, texture, and **price**. Yes! Even the whole grain organic oats that I use is cheaper than any processed packaged cereal. And it only takes minutes to cook! About the same time as toasting two pieces of Vogel's bread.

LOL.

If you are worried about the time it takes to make it, soak it over night that will speed up the cooking time. The oats in grain are energizing while the straw is sedating. Native to northern Europe oats have been cultivated since classical times as early as 2000 B.C. This ancient cereal grass was a staple food for northern Europeans and the Scots. It is also an important food for livestock. Oats are grown commercially from seed, in cooler areas of Australia and New Zealand.

They are high in fibre and protein including amino acids, and low in calories and fat.

Vitamins: A, C and B complex, including thiamine, riboflavin, niacin, folic acid, B6, E and K. Minerals: Silicon, calcium, iron, potassium and phosphorus.

Oats are widely used in human foods, animal feeds and livestock forages around the world. Tinctures and extracts of oat straw are readily available in Europe as a nervous system restorative, to assist convalescence and to strengthen a weakened constitution.

Oat straw is also used in Europe to treat shingles, herpes zoster, herpes simplex and neurasthenia.

Green oat grass (the grass before it matures into oat straw), is rich in vitamins including A, B, C, E, K and pantothenic acid and minerals, including iron (39mg/Kg dry weight), manganese (8.5mg) and zinc (19.2mg), silicon dioxide (2%), calcium, magnesium, phosphorus and potassium.

Green oat grass (14) juice can be used to treat debility. Studies have been conducted on oat grass extract - researchers discovered an influence of the herb on reproductive hormones, including luteinizing hormone.

Perhaps that explains the old saying 'to sow your wild oats'.

This abundance of nutrients has made oat grass a popular tonic for treating debility and convalescence when taken as a juice. Oat grass is also extremely rich in antioxidants, including polyphenols and one powerful antioxidant called tricin.

Current research on oats focuses on the compound, beta-glucan that has been shown to stimulate the immune system. Oat-straw is a cardio-tonic. Good for heart function. As well as an antidepressant that restores the nervous system. Oat straw is cleansing and detoxifying, anti-aging and an antioxidant which stimulates cellular regeneration.

Externally where there is dry skin, burns, itching, hives, eczema and wounds, oats are high in silica so aid skin, hair, connective tissue, muscle tone and function, and local tissue healing.

To summarize, green oat grass is rich in protein, approximately 30%, and contains all the essential amino acids along with chlorophyll, flavonoids, lecithin and enzymes.

OATSTRAW SILICA

To make a decoction and obtain the silica, take one handful of Oat-straw, place in a pot with 1 litre of water and bring to the boil. Reduce heat and simmer for 20 minutes.

For a good winter fortifying drink try oat-straw decoction, a teaspoon of grated fresh ginger root, lemon juice and honey to taste.

Consider a combination of oats and oat-straw for your very own home made body cream - a decoction of oats blended with one or two drops of your favourite essential oil or dried and ground herbs. Try chamomile, mint, pineapple sage, thyme, lavender and dried orange peel, lemon peel, cloves, star anise and blend with an aqueous cream base, to a desired consistency.

Or mix and match ground up dried herbs and dried oats to make an aromatic bath bag and bathe in the beneficial mix.

Refined Grains

Avoid any refined grains. This includes white flour, white rice etc. Wheat allergies(15) are very common these days and responsible for congested air ways as well as:

Swelling, itching or irritation of the mouth or throat.

Hives, itchy rash or swelling of the skin.

Nasal congestion.

Headache.

Itchy, watery eyes.

Difficulty breathing.

Cramps, nausea or vomiting.

Diarrhoea.

What Is White Food?

White food generally refers to foods processed and refined. They are white in colour like flour, rice, pasta, bread, crackers, cereal, and simple sugars like table sugar and high-fructose corn syrup.

Natural, unprocessed white foods, such as onions, white beans, cauliflower, turnips, and white potatoes don't fall into the same category.

The difference between refined white foods and their healthier counterparts is fibre and in the processing. Most white carbohydrates start with flour that has been ground and refined by stripping off the outer layer, where the fibre is located. Vitamins and/or minerals are frequently added back to enrich the refined product. 650 million tons of wheat flour is produced every year in the world today.

The process can be seen in this diagram

'Bad Carbs' Are Less Satisfying (16)

In addition to being easy to overeat, refined carbs are less satisfying than "good carbs." The body absorbs processed grains and simple sugars relatively quickly. Increased blood sugar triggers a release of insulin and, in an hour or two after eating, you're hungry again.

Also, many refined-carb foods - particularly sweetened beverages like fizzy drinks - provide little nutritional value other than calories.

Less processed "good carbs" are higher in volume and tend to be more filling than refined foods.

And controlling portions -- and ultimately, your weight -- is easier when you choose foods that are unprocessed and filling. By making your daily grain servings organic whole grains, you will meet your fibre needs and slow down absorption which will keep you feeling full for much longer.

Some days my porridge for breakfast can keep me going until about 2pm before I even think of eating again.

But keep in mind that not all whole grains are a good source of fibre. For example, brown rice is more nutritious than white rice because it contains the whole kernel of rice, but it's not necessarily the greatest source of fibre.

One thing I am very much in favour of is the abundance of ancient grains on the market now.

Once you have tasted these delicious nutty ancient grains you will not want to have anything else. They are full of nutrition and thousands of years of human consumption. So include plenty of spelt, amaranth, quinoa, millet and kamut in your diet from now on.

5 Ancient Grains

If you haven't tried ancient grains then you are in for a festive explosion of naturally sweet nutty nutrient packed goodness that I am certain once tasted, you will be hooked on.

In addition to offering a higher amount of nutrients and protein than other grains, ancient grains (also called heritage grains) are delicious in taste and can be added to a variety of meals. The rise in popularity in recent years is due to the heightened food sensitivities experienced by what seems to be more and more and more people as well as those who wish to become healthy.

Some of the most popular ancient grains include:

1. Amaranth

Amaranth is often called a "pseudo-grain" and has been referred to as both an herb and a vegetable. However you classify it, amaranth is gluten free and has an impressive nutritional profile, being high in both protein and the amino acid lysine (which is often found in only low amounts in cereal grains). It is also high in fibre and has been shown to be beneficial in lowering cholesterol.

How to prepare:

You will need quite a bit of water when cooking amaranth:

6 cups (1.5 L) of water for 1 cup (250 mL) of amaranth.

Gently boil the amaranth for 15 to 20 minutes, rinse and then fluff it.

Amaranth can be added to soups, salads and stir-fries, and amaranth flour can be used in baking.

2. Kamut

Kamut has 30% more protein than wheat but has less fibre and an excellent alternative to traditional wheat. Originally from Egypt it is a long grain very similar to brown rice. For those

people with an allergy to wheat, kamut can be better tolerated but still requires some caution and is not really tolerated by any one suffering from Celiac disease.

Kamut is also high in selenium, giving this grain strong antioxidant properties, which help protect the immune system. Also known to have a natural sweetness making it a great grain for baking.

How to prepare:

When cooking kamut, it is best to soak the grain overnight. Use three parts water for one part kamut. Once the water has come to a boil, reduce the heat and allow the grain to simmer for 30 to 40 minutes, depending on the tenderness you prefer.

3. Quinoa pronounced: (keen wah)

Quinoa is actually a seed, not a grain. It has gained enormous popularity thanks to its high protein levels (it is a complete protein containing all nine essential amino acids), and because quinoa is gluten free it is a perfect option for those who are sensitive to gluten or have celiac disease.

The seeds are coated with a bitter resin like soapy compound called saponin.

Saponins are phytochemicals (plant chemicals) which have anti – inflammatory, antifungal, antimicrobial and hepato-protective (protects the liver) effects on the body.

When taken orally the therapeutic action of saponins in the digestive tract increases and accelerates the body's ability to absorb some active components e.g. Calcium and silica from foods. They generally assist digestion and help remove cholesterol and other pathogens from your body safely through the digestive tract.

This in turn relieves stress on your immune system allowing it to function more effectively.

Saponins can also relieve eczema and skin allergies, reduce your bone loss and lower your risk of getting various heart diseases and cancers.

How to prepare:

The seeds are prepared similarly to rice and cook very quickly – in about 15 minutes.

Measure one part quinoa to two parts water.

Bring to the boil, lower the heat and allow the quinoa to simmer for 12 to 15 minutes or until the germ separates from the seed (it will look like a little curly tail on the kernel).

Remove the pot from the heat and let stand and absorb the remaining liquid before fluffing the quinoa with a fork.

Cooked quinoa is excellent in casseroles, soups, stews and stir-fries, and is also great cold in salads.

TIP: Instead of cooking grains in just water try infusions of nutritious herbs (Ginger, Rosemary, Sage, Thyme, Mint, Chamomile, Lemon balm and lemongrass just to name a few) to add even more nutrient value:

2 square inches of thinly sliced fresh Ginger would add a warming zing to any grain, a squeeze of lemon and a handful of fresh mint would infuse some amazing flavour and medicinal value.

Use whatever herbs you have at hand.

4. Spelt

Spelt our final ancient grain has been consumed for approximately 9000 years. And until the end of the 19th century accounted for approximately 94% of the cereal acreage compared to wheat at just 5%.

Spelt's fall from popularity coincided with modern farming methods. Once combine harvesters were introduced which could harvest wheat in a single process it would no longer be attractive for farmers to continue to grow spelt.

This is because each individual grain of spelt unlike common wheat is covered by a tough outer husk which requires removal in a further process before the grain can be milled into flour.

Unlike other grains Spelt's goodness is on the inside packed with more protein, fats and crude fibre than wheat and also large amounts of Vitamin B17 (anti-carcinoma). It also contains special carbohydrates which play a decisive role in blood clotting and stimulating the body's immune system so as to increase its resistance to infection.

Also known as Triticum Spelta, spelt is a tasty whole grain with a nutty flavour. This distant cousin of wheat contains gluten and is therefore not suitable for those who have gluten intolerance, it does tend to be easier to digest than wheat and may be better tolerated by those who have a wheat sensitivity.

The real beauty of spelt is in its ability to make a really light, highly nutritious loaf with an appealing nutty flavour. The protein in spelt is such that when the flour is turned into bread it bakes well and results in a very light, soft textured loaf with good keeping qualities which doesn't shed crumbs when sliced. You can use spelt flour in baking, and the grain can be found in a variety of products, including cereals, breads, pasta and crackers.

How to prepare:

Use spelt as you would use regular wheat flour, but be careful with the addition of any liquid portion of a recipe as spelt tends to need slightly less.

Where can I buy my 5 ancient grains?

In most bulk food sections of health stores and organic groceries stores. At this stage not commonly found in Supermarkets, but watch out for them, once a Supermarket finds a popular food, they will definitely stock it.

CHAPTER 3

This chapter is all about the supermarket and the role it has played in changing our lives forever. Allowing a freedom never before experienced in human history. Introducing access to food varieties and preparation methods that would revolutionize the way we live.

Supermarkets

Warning: When you go to the supermarket shop around the outside which is where you will find the majority of your basics - only venture down the aisles for what is absolutely necessary.

Supermarkets and the invention of the home freezer has taken care of the time consuming preparation our grandmothers had in feeding their family.

With more time on her hands the modern mother could consider entering the workforce. Thanks to the supermarket and one stop shopping she was able to buy easy nutritious meals 'TV dinners' to store in the freezer.

Mum no longer had to bottle fruit and vegetables, make jams and marmalade, biscuits, cakes or any other home baking. The supermarket played a critical role in liberating women from the kitchen and into the workforce.

And in today's world it is common and considered essential for families to have both parents working to manage the household budget.

In New Zealand the first supermarket opened in Otahuhu Auckland in 1958.

The Foodtown 'all convenience' store offered 'one stop shopping' selling meat and produce and other grocery items. Most kiwis did their shopping on an as required basis at the corner dairy, the butcher and the green grocer successively.

Only around 54% of kiwis owned a freezer at that time but this was soon to grow. By 1963 we had our second all convenience store 'New World' an American style full service supermarket. And by the late 60s early 70s more Kiwis had a home freezer and were able to shop once a week.

In the early 1970's the supermarket really was an established part of life in most cities in New Zealand. Rural towns would eventually catch up with this trend.

I can remember shopping with my mother, we lived in a small NZ town with no supermarket so it was a trip to the butcher, and the local green grocer who provided almost as much as a supermarket back then without the fancy trimmings. Mums idea of convenience food was the ready- made sponge roll filled with raspberry jam. A slice of sponge roll topped with a tinned apricot and juice with whipped cream.

Walla!

Instant dessert!

But mum was a professional cook all of her meals were prepared from scratch although included in the grocery list were new items like frozen vegetables.

Sixty years ago, Swanson introduced its frozen "TV dinners" and forever changed the family meal.

I was unaware of frozen dinners until the early 1970s.

TV advertising really promoted 'TV dinners' as nutritious, low cost, time saving convenience food and the industry really took off.

Nestle was one of the pioneers of 'TV dinners' growing into a real leader in the industry controlling the biggest share of the freezer space in North American supermarkets.

"We think it is the most exciting thing that has ever happened in the food business," Alan MacDonald, president of Stouffer's, told The New York Times in 1982.

Nestle was one of the pioneers of 'TV dinners' growing into a real leader in the industry controlling the biggest share of the freezer space in North American supermarkets.

"We think it is the most exciting thing that has ever happened in the food business," Alan MacDonald(17), president of Stouffer's, told The New York Times in 1982.

Sales were booming so Nestle and its competitors steadily raised their prices and this worked well until 2008 when the recession hit consumer's pockets hard. No longer able to afford such cuisine, cash-strapped consumers started cooking more from fresh ingredients and saving leftovers for lunch, cutting into sales of frozen meals.

Consumers who were now cooking meals from scratch rapidly discovered they not only saved more money, it tasted so much better and they knew what was going into every meal.

Now they could also avoid the long list of preservatives and salt in frozen dinners which had become a growing concern in the health industry.

Eric Decker(18), head of the food science department at the University of Massachusetts Amherst reveals a long and scary number of preservatives, like calcium propionate, sodium tripolyphosphate, potassium sorbate and ascorbic acid.

Another concern was the amount of salt in prepared meals. Early versions of lean cuisine meals averaged 1000 milligrams of sodium, which is 2/3 the recommended daily allowance for an adult.

The sodium levels have been almost halved now and Nestle have pledged to reduce sodium slowly and steadily by a further 10 per cent by 2015.

While Nestle spokesperson Roz O'Hearn(19) said, Nestle frozen foods use "the same quality ingredients our consumers purchase when cooking from scratch".

Consumers are not convinced and have been reducing consumption of frozen meals on an increasing basis since 2008.

Sales are down by a quarter in the last 5 years according to researcher Mintel.

Today's consumer is well aware that frozen dinners offer no or little nutritional value, they cost more and are unhealthy no matter how many discounts and competitions are offered with their meals, sales are steadily declining.

"It's a health and wellness issue, not just an economic one," said <u>Alexia Howard</u>(20), an analyst at Sanford C Bernstein. "The category is not coming back no matter how heavily they promote it."

Some frozen meals however have increased in sales and those that have been successful promote a healthier alternative.

Amy's Kitchen's organic, offer vegetarian meals like black bean veggie enchiladas and sales have increased by 13 per cent to US$240m in the year ended February 25, according to Nielsen. Hillshire Brands, a meat business spun out of Sara Lee, will take its Jimmy Dean brand beyond breakfast this year with smoked bacon mac & cheese.

Iglo Group, Europe's biggest frozen-food company, is helping retailers redesign freezer aisles to look like restaurants or fish markets.

"People want to be inspired to eat food, not a bag of ice," said Iglo Chief executive Elio Leoni Sceti.

Sixty years ago, Swanson introduced its frozen "TV dinners" and forever changed the family meal.

Sixty years on, today's consumer is more informed with the dangers of preservatives in food and looks for a healthier alternative preferring fresh ingredients which they have discovered is cheaper than frozen packaged meals and healthier too.

What are the future trends in supermarket shopping?

According to a recent FMI annual survey today's shopper is more likely to 'channel surf' exploring the options available rather than rely solely on what's in their local supermarket. It is also more likely the shopping is split with men now accounting for more than 40% of primary shoppers. There is also a generational transformation, 50+ shoppers tend to shop once a week, but the millennial generation are more spontaneous and tend to purchase meals they will consume that day.

Health and wellness is emerging as the most important factor in today's shopper, 92% believe eating at home is healthier than eating out. And finally the report shows today's shopper is interested in the supermarket becoming more personable trusted allies in their wellbeing.

According to data, 43% of all shoppers view their primary store as a trusted source of healthy food and wellness. The supermarket of the future will have to engage the customer in a more personal way, tips and meal suggestions, discounting deals, loyalty deals and rewards for example.

My supermarket has a loyalty card which gives them a record of everything I buy and when something I buy comes up on special they let me know.

It has all become so sophisticated.

The range of foods to choose from has also grown. New and exotic choices fill the supermarket shelves enticing you to try them. In the past 40 or so years our traditional diet has changed considerably. Did you know by consuming a more traditional diet you are less likely to have digestive problems. When we look at foods such as spelt, a food which had been consumed in huge numbers for 9000 years right up until the 19th century, our experience of consuming wheat is put into perspective.

Preserved and packaged food has entered our busy lives to help save us time and energy, but at what cost?

Most supermarkets are set up in the same way. When the shopper enters the supermarket, the first isle is generally where the fresh fruit and vegetables are. Many of the fruit and vegetables we have available in the supermarket are chosen for their uniform shape and appearance as well as its shelf life rather than its nutritional value. Large commercial growers look for these qualities when considering what to plant. And while the supermarket may promote their produce as fresh, the reality is this is not always the case. Most supermarkets use a centralized buying centre where produce is freighted long distances from where it has been grown. Food miles and fuel costs significantly add to the total cost of the product and this is passed on to the consumer. Freshness is also affected, supermarkets will import produce when local supplies are scarce, but the cost is high and the eating quality poor. For example, NZ apples in winter are excellent value for money and top quality, whereas apples imported from the USA in summer can be expensive and of disappointing quality. We've all bought that delicious looking apple and while they look great, once you bite into the apple it lacks freshness and can be floury or even rotten, very disappointing. We are also missing out on so many more varieties of heritage fruit and vegetables that are steadily disappearing.

"Did you know that a large proportion of the heritage fruit and vegetables on the planet have either passed into extinction or are rapidly headed that way"?

We live in an age in which we're rapidly losing traditional knowledge. Many of the handy, practical things our parents and grandparents knew about the world have been lost".

These heritage plants pack more nutritional value than anything you can buy on a supermarket shelf. *Where possible buy heritage seeds and grow your own fruit and vegetables, you will definitely notice the difference they are packed with flavour and nutrition".*

Visit:

http://www.koanga.org.nz

CHAPTER 4

Chapter four is all about the farmers market and how they are helping to revitalize the food we eat by providing home made locally produced fresh products.

Farmers Markets

The growth in the farmers markets around New Zealand is no surprise. Small local enterprises can set up a stall and sell local produce directly to the public. They fill the consumer's needs by providing accurate information about the product directly from the person who knows best the producer.

Consumers are aware of the origin of the product, how best to use it, store it and consume it. Consumers can build a strong trusting and valued relationship with the producer and any problems can be dealt with face to face.

The producer benefits from feedback, praise, suggestions and loyalty from their customer.

Health conscious kiwis are looking for organic foods free from chemicals, pesticides, hormones and antibiotics at the best price possible and the farmers market is an excellent source of organic and truly fresh food. The low overheads and absence of the middle man makes for cheaper prices and fresher produce that has often been picked that very same day.

Choices are also affected with the consumer able to purchase exclusive local specialty foods, vegetables, oils, meats, herbs and items that don't store or transport well such as heirloom fruit and vegetables that are not stocked in supermarkets. More variety in the diet ensures more nutrients consumed.

The people who enjoy selling their produce often have more passion and help to generate interest in home cooked meals often passing on favourite recipes and tips for customers who enjoy trying new foods. Which in turn reduces consumption of processed convenience foods.

Some regional specialties like Bluff Oysters, Pokeno Bacon and Central Otago apricots also provide a public awareness and pride in their community. Increased support of farmers markets will encourage producers to try new varieties and provide more choice than the 'repetitiveness' of supermarket produce. Some products, by cutting out the middle man are well priced and a fairer price for the producer and customer alike.

Everyone benefits!

Consumers are becoming more aware of the cost of fuel these days and the affect it is having on our wallets. Most of us shop at the supermarket and the cost of food must contain these prices.

These food miles account for much of the cost of the item to the consumer. Awareness is growing about the effect on our environment and more sustainable practices within the community and supported within the community will bring these costs down.

Another danger we face these days which must be considered is genetically modified foods. The risk is real but impossible to calculate for consumers because processed foods contain a large variety of ingredients from many sources while the food may contain canola oil imported from the US this may not appear on the labelling.

Most Canola oil from the USA is from genetically modified crops.

Buying locally made produce will ensure there is no possibility of consuming any GE foods.

Smaller enterprises using sustainable practices can produce a wide range of crops and animal foods that have been nurtured in a carefully managed natural environment.

They can tell you exactly what pest control has been used and when or if any has been used. And because the consumer is buying locally and seasonally they are assured of the very best price.

The consumer that buys locally from small producers help support their local communities, they increase awareness and pride in local products and help regenerate a sense of kinship.

While they may not be able to compete with some imported items which are cheaper e.g.: (tomatoes from Australia imported in our off season) they certainly can compete with freshness, nutrient value, local knowledge, local wealth, "localization" and relationships. As opposed to the supermarket equivalent of questionable or unknown ingredients, salt, sugar, preservatives, GE foods, plastics, packaging and obstruction of local small business.

Your food choices are paramount to your wellness, reducing questionable produce from the supermarket and increasing locally made produce is sure to maximize your health as well as You're community's wealth.

CHAPTER 5

The traditional diet and the benefits of eating the food our ancestors ate.

A Traditional Diet.

There are many Traditional Diets.

Dr Weston A. Price's (21) travelled around the world in the early 1900's, to study Traditional diets in detail. These cultures all ate quite differently. Some ate no plant foods, some ate a lot. Some ate dairy, some did not. The variations in diet are vast and go on and on. The common denominator between these cultures is that they all had at least one sacred food which was **always from an animal**, and not from plants.

These sacred foods were discovered in laboratory analysis to be extraordinary high in the fat soluble vitamins A, D, and K2.

And what is extraordinary is that these Traditional Cultures were consuming the fat soluble activators at a rate about 10x higher than we do today. These sacred foods were revered by the Traditional

Cultures that consumed them for bestowing easy fertility and healthy babies.

Ample quantities of these sacred foods were provided to growing children, pregnant mothers, and the elderly to maintain health and the prevention of tooth decay. With so many different Traditional Diets, you can see why it's important to investigate your own unique genetic heritage.

This was a surprise to me when I studied nutrition. To find out that what I thought I was eating was good for me was incorrect.

It turns out that mum's meat and three veg was actually a better diet for me and more in tune with my unique genetic heritage.

My Traditional Diet could easily be misconstrued by some, as the way to eat traditionally, when it is, in fact, only the implementation of a mix of Traditional Diets that work for me given my unique genetic heritage, health history, home environment, toxin load, food budget and so on.

So! How to Determine the Best Traditional Diet for YOU

Research has shown that traditional diets (22) around the world protect ethnic folk from the major killer diseases-cancer and atherosclerosis—which have become rampant in the industrialized world. Should we, therefore, track down our genetic lineage and adopt the diet of our great-grandparents? Well that's almost correct.

First of all. What is YOUR Ancestral Heritage?

When you take a look at your genetic heritage and focus your Traditional Diet on those foods consumed by your specific culture and ancestors. In most cases we are such a genetic mix of cultures that it is hard to pin down exactly what to eat. However thankfully, many of these traditional diets have some foods in common.

Therefore I would look for: Natural whole foods which are locally and seasonally available.

This is very important, as you may note we tend to grow root vegetables in winter and leafy greens or above ground vegetables in summer.

Foods that are high in enzymes, either because they are fresh and raw or because they have been naturally preserved through traditional fermentation methods and natural, unrefined fats such as butter, flaxseed oil, olive oil and coconut oil.

You also should consider that you live in a different climate and environment. You are likely to be less physically active than your ancestors, even if you exercise regularly. This means that you should eat fewer acid-forming foods such as meat and more alkaline-forming foods such as fruit and vegetables, which also supply plenty of enzymes when eaten raw.

It is also safe to eat traditionally fermented foods?

Traditionally Fermented Foods

Lactic-acid fermented foods, for instance, are partially pre-digested through enzyme action. Yogurt, kefir and buttermilk are lactic-acid fermented dairy foods which have traditionally been consumed by ethnic groups known for their extraordinary sturdiness and longevity.

Although mandatory pasteurization and homogenization have robbed us of the benefits of enzyme-rich raw milk and dairy products, we can still enjoy cultured milk products in which enzyme action is restored. People of different ethnic backgrounds who are unable to digest regular milk find that fermented milks give them no such problems. The health benefits of natural fermentation are also known in traditional Asian cuisine, where cultured soy products such as miso, tempeh and natto are popular. Many vegetables can be lactic-acid fermented, including cabbage (the sauerkraut of northern and eastern Europe), carrots, radishes, cucumbers, tomatoes and beets.

Traditionally, sauerkraut is prepared by shredding and mashing the veggies to squeeze out the juice, mixing the pulp and juice with salt and water, then packing everything tightly in a Mason jar and allowing it to stand at room temperature for several days.

The naturally present lactic-acid bacteria then initiates the fermentation process, converting the sugars and starches into lactic acid, which helps to restore a healthy bowel flora and destroys putrefactive bacteria in the intestines.

Commercially prepared lactic-acid fermented vegetables are available in many natural food stores. Be sure to buy an unpasteurized product.

Unless specific intolerances are present, these foods are nourishing and health-giving for people of all ethnic backgrounds.

Soaking and Sprouting

Many traditional diets also rely on soaking, sprouting and sour-leavening to make foods more nutritious and easier to digest.

These practices help to break down the phytates in grains and seeds, which otherwise interfere with the absorption of minerals in the body.

Sprouting also multiplies the vitamin content of plant foods.

What traditional diets lack is refined flour and sugar, overcooked foods devoid of enzymes, pasteurized milk and cheese and processed, hydrogenated vegetable oils. When our digestive system revolts and we find that we can no longer tolerate certain grains or dairy, it is not necessarily because these foods were absent from our great-grandparents' diet. But rather, it is the modern, processed versions of these foods which are indigestible and cause illness.

Whatever your ancestral lineage is, you will benefit if you put the enzyme-rich, unrefined organic whole foods of traditional diets back into daily diet from now on!

Why These Diets Work

The late Dr Weston A. Price, concluded from his research that it was largely the abundance of the fat-soluble vitamins A and D in native diets that determined the overall nutritional status and health of the natives.

Dr Price found that ethnic groups who changed their diet from native food to imported modern foods then suffered rampant tooth decay, which led to other health problems (toothache was the only cause of suicide among natives of Fiji, for example).

The new generation whose parents adopted processed foods had crowded teeth and changes in the shape of the face and dental arches.

This can be apparent today when we look at the generally soft pallor of many of our children. Children today in the western world are also more obese, compare that with their grandparents and great grandparents and you will note that we have got much bigger than our ancestors.

Also in the last century, physician Dr Edward Howell, the author of *Enzyme Nutrition*, spent many years researching the health benefit of enzyme-rich raw foods in ethnic diets and human nutrition. He concluded that enzymes in a natural foods diet are the vital link in the digestion and assimilation of foods and in preventing chronic degenerative disease and premature death.

Lipase, the enzyme necessary for fat digestion, is abundantly available in un-pasteurized dairy products and is important for the proper assimilation of vitamins A and D from these foods.

The Most Important Key to Implementation of Traditional Diet.

Is to focus on what was considered common foods consumed by your ancestors.

Eat plenty of **these critical foods!**

Also eat what is in season. To help aid digestion include traditionally fermented foods, especially if you tend to have food allergies.

And as always, **"Fresh is Best Forget the Rest"**.

To ensure maximum health and immunity to disease both infectious and chronic.

CHAPTER 6

The food we eat is paramount to our health. So is the environment we live in. In this chapter we look at the chemicals in house hold cleaners. List some alternatives. And look at some of the things we wouldn't normally take any notice of.

10 dangerous things in modern homes

1/ Bread

There is nothing like the smell of freshly cooked bread however not everyone enjoys the after effects of eating bread. Gluten is a mixture of two proteins present in cereal grains, including wheat, which is responsible for the elastic texture and structure of dough. People barely talked about gluten 10 years ago, there has always been people with a gluten intolerance, but not as many as there seems to be today. Now everyone has heard of 'gluten free food' and it appears to be a growing industry.

It must be!

We see it in the supermarket.

Entire areas dedicated to gluten free food. Is this because more people are intolerant or is it because gluten free menus are all the rage, people who are influenced by the benefits of 'gluten free' which is said to contribute to increased energy, thinner thighs, and reduced belly bloating would flock to have a product like this.

Unless you are genuinely gluten intolerant you stand to miss out on some vital nutrients. Many people may just perceive that a gluten-free diet is healthier.

The fact is it isn't.

For people with celiac disease, a gluten-free diet is essential. But for others, "unless people are very careful, a gluten-free diet can lack vitamins, minerals, and fibre.

Avoiding these foods means saying no to many vital nutrients that need to be replaced.

"And any time you eliminate whole categories of food you've been used to eating, you run the risk of nutritional deficiencies," said Green.

A 2005 report from the American Dietetic Association warned that gluten-free products tend to be low in a wide range of important nutrients, including B vitamins, calcium, iron, zinc, magnesium, and fibre.

If you are not gluten intolerant and want to avoid gluten the safest way is to incorporate foods high in vitamins, minerals and fibre a few whole grains that don't contain gluten, are amaranth, millet, and quinoa.

2/ Milk

Lactose intolerance - People with lactose intolerance may feel uncomfortable 30 minutes to 2 hours after consuming milk, cheese and milk products. Symptoms range from mild to severe, based on the amount of lactose consumed and the amount a person can tolerate.

Common symptoms include: abdominal pain, abdominal bloating, cramps, diarrhoea and nausea.

People with lactose intolerance just don't have enough lactase the enzyme that breaks down the lactose sugars in the digestive tract. The important thing to know here is that lactose intolerance has nothing to do with having a milk allergy, they are quite different.

The Symptoms of a true milk allergy include a skin rash, vomiting, runny nose, puffy eyes, difficulty breathing and tightness in the throat. To ensure you are getting your daily allowance of calcium if you are lactose intolerant is to eat plenty of green vegetables.

And the very best way is to take probiotics. Yoghurts and probiotics help reduce symptoms by slowing down the digestive process, introducing beneficial bacteria to help digestion and reducing your sensitivity to the symptoms.

3/ Sugar

Sugar is a naked carbohydrate – refined sugar consumption has increased 10 fold in 150 years. The majority of people eat their weight in sugar each year. Problem is sugar is also hidden most packaged and tinned foods. The food industry has 56 different names for sugar so read your labels carefully.

Sometimes disguised as 'energy'.

The metabolism of sugar will only proceed through the use of all accessory nutrients which are involved in its combustion. Which means when sugar is taken into the body nutrients: vitamins, minerals, fats and proteins must be pulled from any body tissue or organs to enable the body to process it. And when large quantities of refined sugar are eaten the body becomes increasingly deficient in important nutrients and stores it in fat tissue for later assimilation.

4/ Vitamin Supplements

Evidence from studies of almost half a million people suggested that "supplementing the diet of well-nourished adults... has no clear benefit and might even be harmful (23)", despite one in three Britons taking vitamins or mineral pills. The conclusions were drawn by academics from the University of Warwick and the Johns Hopkins School of Medicine in Baltimore, the US, and published in the Annals of Internal Medicine. The scientists also suggested that companies selling supplements were fuelling false health anxieties to offer unnecessary cures,

The Times said. On analysing 24 previous trials involving 450,000 people, found no beneficial effect on mortality from taking vitamins. Another examined 6,000 elderly men and found no improvement on cognitive decline after 12 years of taking supplements, while a third saw no advantage of supplements among 1,700 men and women with heart problems over an average study of five years.

The experts said most supplements should be avoided as their use is not justified, writing:

"These vitamins should not be used for chronic disease prevention. Enough is enough."

They said that an average Western diet is sufficient to provide the necessary vitamins the body needs". This is an interesting argument because on one hand they are saying the food available to us is nutrient poor? Yet on the other hand we are told the average western diet is nutrient rich? How do we answer this question?

"The whole is greater than the sum of its parts".

If you are going to take supplements perhaps it is best to take them in their whole food form. Whole herb extracts, seaweed products, flax seed oil and coconut oil would fit the bill.

5/ All Weight Loss Diets

Many weight loss diet taken long-term can be harmful as they tend to exclude important nutrients and important food groups. The safest diet to follow is "fresh is best forget the rest" which means butter is better than margarine, whole foods from natures garden fresh fruit and vegetables, fresh meat not packaged or processed is best. Our bodies recognize these foods and metabolize them efficiently.

6/Asbestos.

Significant exposure to any type of asbestos will increase the risk of lung cancer, and non-malignant lung and pleural disorders, including asbestosis, pleural plaques, pleural thickening, and pleural effusions.

This conclusion is based on observations of these diseases in groups of workers with cumulative exposures ranging from about 5 to 1,200 fibre year/ml.

Asbestos can be found in your own home, in brake pads, automobile clutches, roofing materials, vinyl tile and imported cement pipe and corrugated sheeting. Until the 1970s, asbestos was widely used in the construction, shipbuilding, mining and automotive industries.

7/ Insulation.

Over a million New Zealander's still live in damp and draughty houses. The World Health Organisation research shows that if your home is constantly below 18 degrees C, you are much more at risk from colds, bronchitis or asthma. One in six New Zealand adults and one in four children experience asthma symptoms.

These are some of the highest rates in the world. Effective house insulation pays immediate dividends. A University of Otago study has shown that improving the home environment through insulation and heating cut hospital admissions for respiratory conditions by 38%. As a bonus, energy use was reduced by 19%.

8/ Mold.

Exposure to damp and moldy environments may cause a variety of health effects, or none at all. Some people are sensitive to molds. For these people, molds can cause nasal stuffiness, throat irritation, coughing or wheezing, eye irritation, or, in some cases, skin irritation. People with mold allergies may have more severe reactions. Immune-compromised people and people with chronic lung illnesses, such as obstructive lung disease, may get serious infections in their lungs when they are exposed to mold.

These people should stay away from areas that are likely to have mold, such as compost piles, cut grass, and wooded areas. In 2004 the Institute of Medicine (IOM) found there was sufficient evidence to link indoor exposure to mold with upper respiratory tract symptoms, cough, and wheeze in otherwise healthy people with asthma symptoms in people with asthma; and with hypersensitivity pneumonitis in individuals susceptible to that immune-mediated condition. The IOM also found limited or suggestive evidence linking indoor mold exposure and respiratory illness in otherwise healthy children.

9/ **Bottled Water**

I have actually bought bottled water on a couple of occasions. Madness!

The power of advertising eh!

I have bought bottled water so I'm a contributor to the plastic that ends up on our beaches all over the world. I don't even have a good excuse because I can get perfectly good drinking water from my tap. We have local councils that have stringent rules to abide by to make sure we get the very best drinking water. My sister-in-law who lives in Australia can't get enough of our tap water. When she comes to NZ and raves about it. When bottled water first came out I thought this will not catch on but it has and here we are enveloped in a mountain of plastic.

Some bottled water comes in glass bottles but the majority is plastic. Is it actually any better? Try the taste test, see if you can taste the chlorine? In most cases the source of the water needs to be considered, e.g.: the condition of the pipes to your tap.

Most tap water contains chlorine to kill bacteria and fluoride for healthy teeth. Whoever came up with the idea is simply genius because I can't think of a better sham.

10/ *Plastics*

Over just a few decades man-made plastics have found their way into the ocean. Plastics take thousands of years to decay. Fish and wildlife are affected. Toxins from plastics have entered the food chain also threatening human health. Samples taken from remote beaches 28% of samples sifted were found to be plant material, fragments of mollusk shells or large grains of sand and 70% of the sample collected was plastics.

This is horrific!

It is bad enough we contaminate our own back yard but the fact we contaminate the entire planet is unforgiveable.

A solution has been found and actually known about for some time, only it wasn't really viable until now.

It's brilliant really 'killing two birds with one stone' (metaphor wouldn't really do it) called Air Carbon.

New-light technologies (24) have perfected it, pulling carbon emissions from the atmosphere and turning it into plastic. Recycling if you will but out of the atmosphere and into your next car, cellphone cases, lunch box, other food containers, bottled water! The list goes on.

HOME MADE NON TOXIC HOUSEHOLD CLEANERS

Today's modern home is loaded with toxic and polluting substances designed to make domestic life easier.

The cost of these commercial, chemical based products can be high with long term health concerns for the family and environmental pollution caused by their manufacture and disposal.

Should any member of your family suffer from allergies, asthma, sinusitis or bronchitis, treatment for these conditions should include reducing synthetic chemicals in the home environment.

For many home cleaning chores, you can make your own cleaning products using the formulas listed below. A growing number of commercial non-toxic home cleaning products are also available, as healthier and environmentally responsible alternatives.

Your use of these products helps promote the growth of 'Green Businesses' which are contributing to a local sustainable economy.

HOME MADE SUBSTITUTIONS

There are many inexpensive, easy to use, natural alternatives which can safely be used in place of commercial household products. Here is a list of common, environmentally safe products which can be used alone or in combination for a wealth of household applications.

Baking Soda

Cleans, deodorizes, softens water and scours

Soap

Unscented soap in liquid form, flakes, powders or bars, are biodegradable and will clean just about anything.

Avoid using soaps which contain petroleum distillates.

Borax

(Sodium- bicarbonate) cleans, deodorises, disinfects, softens water, cleans wallpaper, painted walls and floors.

White vinegar

Cuts grease, removes mildew, odours, some stains and wax build up.

Washing soda

Cuts grease, removes stains, softens water, cleans walls, tiles, sinks and tubs.

Use with care as washing soda can irritate mucus membranes. Do not use on aluminium.

Corn-starch

Corn-starch can be used to clean windows, polish furniture, shampoo carpets and rugs.

Trisodium phosphate (TSP).

A mixture of soda ash and phosphoric acid. TSP is toxic if swallowed, but it can be used on many jobs, such as cleaning drains or removing old paint. This does not create any fumes.

FORMULAS

Combinations of the above basic products can provide less harmful substitutions for many commercial home products.

In most cases, they are also a lot less expensive. **Here are some formulas:**

These formulas and substitutions are offered to help minimize the use of toxic substances in your home, and reduce the environmental harm caused by the manufacture, use and disposal of toxins.

Results may vary and cannot be guaranteed to be 100% safe and effective.

Before applying any cleaning formulations, test in small hidden areas if possible.

Always use caution with any new product in your home.

Make sure to keep all homemade formulas well-labelled and out of reach of children.

ALL PURPOSE CLEANER

Mix ½ cup of vinegar

¼ cup of baking soda or borax into 2 litres of water.

Keep and store well-labelled. Use for water stains from shower, bathroom chrome, windows, and bathroom mirrors, etc.

Microfiber cloths lift off dirt, grease and dust without the need for cleaning chemicals because they are formulated to penetrate and trap dirt.

There are a number of different brands. A good quality cloth can last for years.

AIR FRESHENER

Commercial air fresheners mask smells and coat nasal passages to diminish the sense of smell.

Baking soda or vinegar with lemon juice in a small dish will absorb odours around the house.

House plants help reduce odours around the home.

Simmering vinegar (1 tsp in 1 cup of water) when cooking will reduce odours.

To get the smell of fish and onion off utensils and cutting boards, wipe them with vinegar and wash in soapy water.

Simmer cinnamon and other spices in water on stove.

Place fragrant flowers and herbs in rooms and place bunches of dried herbs in cupboards for a refreshing scent.

CARPET STAINS

Mix equal parts of white vinegar and water in a spray bottle.

Spray directly on stain, let it sit for several minutes and clean with a brush or sponge using warm soapy water.

For a heavy duty carpet cleaner, mix ¼ cup each of salt, borax and vinegar.

Rub into a paste place on area and leave to dry and vacuum off.

DISHWASHER SOAP

Mix equal parts of borax and washing soda, but increase the washing soda if your water is hard.

DISHWASHING SOAP

Commercial low- phosphate detergents are not themselves harmful, but phosphates nourish algae which use up oxygen in the water ways.

A detergent substitution is to use liquid soap.

Add 2 or 3 tablespoons of vinegar to the warm soapy water for tough jobs.

DISINFECTANT

Mix 2 tsp of borax,

4 tbsps. Vinegar

3 cups of hot water.

For stronger cleaning power add ¼ tsp liquid castile soap.

Wipe on with dampened cloth or use a non- aerosol spray bottle.

DRAIN CLEANER

Pour ½ cup baking soda down the drain then ½ cup of vinegar.

The resulting chemical reaction can break down fatty acids into soap and glycerin, allowing the clog to wash away down the drain. After 15 minutes, pour boiling water to clear residue.

Caution: *only use this method with metal pipes as boiling water can melt plastic pipes.*

Also, do not use this method after trying commercial drain cleaner as the vinegar can react with the drain cleaner and create dangerous fumes.

STATIC CLING

To reduce static cling, dampen your hands, and shake out your clothes as you remove them from the drier.

Line drying clothing is the best alternative.

FLOOR CLEANER AND POLISH

Vinyl and linoleum: *add a capful of baby oil to the cleaning water to preserve and polish.*

Wood: *apply a thin coat of 1:1 vegetable oil and vinegar with a few drops of essential oil for aroma and rub in well.*

Painted wood: *mix 1 tsp washing soda into 4 litres of hot water.*

Brick and stone tiles: *Mix 1 cup of white vinegar in 4 litres of water, rinse with clear water.*

Most floor surfaces can be cleaned with equal parts of white distilled vinegar and water with 15 drops of your favourite essential oil - shake and mix.

Furniture polish:

For varnished wood, add a few drops of lemon oil into ½ cup of warm water, spray onto a soft cloth. The cloth should only be slightly damp. Wipe furniture with the cloth using wide strokes to distribute oil evenly.

LAUNDRY DETERGENT

Mix 1 cup of liquid soap, ½ cup washing soda and ½ cup of borax. Use 1 tsp for light loads and 2tsp for heavy loads.

LIME DEPOSITS

You can reduce lime deposits in your tea pot and jug by using ½ cup white vinegar and 2 cups of water, and gently boil for a few minutes.

Rinse well with fresh water while jug is still warm.

METAL CLEANERS AND POLISHERS

Aluminum: *Using a soft cloth, clean with a solution of cream of tartar and water.*

Brass or bronze:

Polish with a soft cloth dipped in lemon juice and baking soda solution, or vinegar and salt solution.

Chrome:

Polish with baby oil, vinegar, or Aluminium foil shiny side out.

Copper:

Soak a cotton rag in a pot of boiling water with 1 tbsp. of salt and 1 cup of white vinegar.

Apply to copper while hot, let it cool, then wipe clean. For tougher jobs, sprinkle baking soda and lemon juice on the cloth before wiping.

Gold:

Clean with toothpaste, or a paste of salt, vinegar and flour.

Silver:

Line a pan with aluminium foil and fill with water, add a tsp each of baking soda and salt.

Bring pan to the boil and immerse the silver. Polish with a soft cloth.

Stainless steel:

Clean with a cloth dampened with undiluted white vinegar.

Mould and mildew:

Use white vinegar or lemon juice full strength, with a small amount of salt.

Apply using a sponge or a spray bottle and do not rinse.

MOTHBALLS

The common mothball is made of <u>paradichlorobenzene (25)</u>, which is harmful to liver and kidneys.

Cedar chips in a cheese-cloth or cedar oil in an absorbent cloth will repel moths. The cedar should be 'aromatic cedar', also referred to as juniper in some areas. Cedar chips are available at many craft supply outfits, or make your own using a plane and a block of cedar from a supplier.

Homemade moth repelling sachets can also be made with lavender and rosemary - you will find that lavender scent in particular will last for decades. Dried lemon peel can also be used simply tossed into a cheese cloth and hung in the closet.

Dried whole orange with cloves pressed into the surface also works well.

OVEN CLEANER

Moisten oven surfaces with a sponge and water. Use ¾ cup of baking soda, ¼ cup salt and ¼ cup of water to make a thick paste, and spread throughout the oven interior (avoid bare metal and any openings), let it sit over-night.

Remove with a spatula and wipe clean.

Rub gently with fine steel wool for stubborn areas.

If you are about my age you will remember 'Chemico(26) '. It was the only oven cleaner available when I was a child; my mum used this pink paste to clean the oven, stainless steel, chrome, enamel baths and basins. This product is still available, does a good job and is fully biodegradable.

PAINT BRUSH CLEANER

Non-toxic citrus oil based solvents are now available under several brands.

This works well for cleaning brushes of oil based paints. Paint brushes and rollers to be used for an ongoing project can be saved overnight, or even up to a week, without cleaning at all simply wrap the brush or roller snugly in a plastic bag, squeeze out air pockets and store away from the light in a dark cupboard.

Fresh paint odours can be reduced by placing a small dish of white vinegar in the room.

PERMANENT INK MARKERS

These markers contain harmful solvents such as toluene, xylene and ethanol.

Use water based markers as a safe substitute.

RUST REMOVER

Sprinkle a little salt on rust, squeeze lime juice over salt until it is well soaked.

Leave the mixture on for 2-3 hours.

Use leftover rind to scrub residue.

SCOURING POWDER

For the top of the stove, refrigerator and other areas which should not be scratched use baking soda. Apply directly with a damp sponge.

SHOE POLISH

Olive oil with a few drops of lemon juice can be applied to shoes with a thick cotton or terry cloth.

Leave for a few minutes, then wipe and buff with a clean dry rag.

TOILET BOWL CLEANER

Mix ¼ cup baking soda and one cup vinegar, pour into basin and let it set for a few minutes.

Scrub with a brush and rinse.

A mixture of borax - 1 part and lemon juice 2 parts will also work.

TUB AND TILE CLEANER

For simple cleaning, rub in baking soda with a damp sponge and rinse with fresh water.

For tougher jobs, wipe surfaces with vinegar first and follow with baking soda as a scouring powder.

(Vinegar can break down tile grout so use sparingly on this surface).

WALLPAPER REMOVER

Mix equal parts of white vinegar and hot water, apply with a sponge over the old wallpaper to soften the adhesive. Open doors and windows or use a fan to dispel the vinegar smell.

WATER RINGS ON WOOD

Water rings on a wooden table or counter are the result of moisture that is trapped under the top coat. Try applying toothpaste or mayonnaise to a damp cloth and rub into the ring. Once the ring is removed, buff the entire wood surface.

WINDOW CLEANER

Mix 2 tsp white vinegar with 1 litre of warm water.

Use crumpled newspaper or a cotton cloth to clean.

Don't clean windows if the sun is on them, or if they are warm, or streaks will show on drying.

The 'All Purpose Cleaner' above also works well on windows. The best product I have found for cleaning windows these days is Kleenex Viva glass and mirror wipes.

The 'woven web' design of the cloth attracts oily residue and marks leaving a streak free and lint free clean using only water.

They're awesome but hard to come by.

When I see them in the supermarket I grab them. Not sure why they are so hard to come by?

But I wouldn't be without them now.

I found they even got rid of the old film left on the windows from products used in the past.

HEALTHY HOME CLEANING HABITS

EXCHANGE AIR

Many modern homes are so tight there's little new air coming in. Open the windows from time to time or run installed exhaust fans. In cold weather, the most efficient way to exchange room air is to open the room wide – (windows and doors) and let fresh air in quickly for about 5 minutes. The furnishings in the room, and the walls, act as 'heat sinks'; and by exchanging the air quickly, this heat is retained.

MINIMIZE DUST

Remove clutter which collects dust, such as old newspapers and magazines. Try to initiate a 'no-shoes-inside' policy. If you are building, consider an inbuilt vacuum system as this eliminates the fine dust which portable vacuum cleaners re-circulate.

KEEP BEDROOMS CLEAN

Often, most time is spent in the bedrooms (you sleep there all night!); keep pets out of these rooms, especially if they spend time outdoors.

USE GENTLE CLEANING PRODUCTS

Of the various commercial home cleaning products, drain cleaners, toilet bowl cleaners and oven cleaners are the most toxic. Use the formulas above or purchase green alternatives.

Avoid products containing ammonia, chlorine, or petroleum based chemicals; these contribute to respiratory irritation, headaches and other complaints.

CLEAN FROM TOP DOWN

When you are house cleaning, save the floor or carpet for last.

Allow time for the dust to settle before vacuuming.

COMMERCIAL NON-TOXIC HOUSEHOLD PRODUCTS

Commercial home-cleaning products are available today which are effective, easy to use and safe for the environment. These natural products can often cost more, but are worth it.

Consider the added cost as an investment in your family's health.

Anyone in your family who suffers from asthma, hay-fever, eczema, sinusitis, dermatitis or bronchitis will thank you.

By removing just some of the more harmful, toxic cleaning products you have in your home at present, you will be helping yourself and your entire family's wellbeing, as well as helping to support businesses which are providing environmentally safe alternatives.

A clean environmentally friendly home is a very good start to improving your health.

Installing a DVS, HRV or other similar system to recycle the hot warm air trapped in your roof will warm your house in winter and cool your house in summer.

It will also circulate air that could become stuffy, help eliminate mould and damp spots and at a relatively low cost.

By drying out a damp house you will reduce heating costs, as heating has to remove the moisture before it can begin to heat your home.

A dehumidifier will also take moisture out of a damp house, in turn reducing the energy it takes to heat your home. Friends have just bought a dehumidifier and were amazed to discover that after placing it in their daughter's bedroom for the first time, they collected 16 litres of water in a very short time. They also noticed the house was at least a few degrees warmer in only a few days of use. Moisture in the home breeds bugs that can also be responsible for many respiratory conditions the family may suffer from.

Every home should have a shower dome - it makes a lot of sense to put a lid on your shower and trap all that moisture in.

Shower domes which can be fitted to most shower boxes save a lot of energy. The shower does not have to be as hot because the air is trapped in the capsule. Therefore you will find you do not turn the tap up quite so high, the bathroom does not steam up and your mirror will remain clear. This means a lot less moisture in your bathroom which can often be a breeding ground for mould. We found after installing a shower dome over 10 years ago our bathroom no longer has problems with mould.

Prior to having the shower dome installed we were regularly painting the bathroom ceiling regardless of using mould repellent paint and it seemed we were always cleaning up mouldy walls. The shower dome saved all of that and another unexpected benefit was the moisture captured in the shower would help self - clean the walls by reducing soap scum.

When we first moved into our home which was built in the 1920's we faced a number of issues. About 2-3 nights after moving in my husband was woken in the night by the sound of dripping water - the header tank in the roof had overflowed. As it turns out this had happened many times before and over the years the overflow tray had rusted out causing water to run into the ceiling and drip, drip, drip onto the dining room floor. Thankfully there was no damage to the ceiling and it was easy to fix.

The next issue was a down pipe at the front of the house which had also rusted out causing water to pool under the house and rot the piles. This would have made the house very damp and cold. Every bedroom in the house had a wall heater and our bedroom was by far the worst.

It smelt musty unless I aired the room daily.

I could not leave anything under the bed or in the wardrobe without it collecting mould over the winter. Shoes would be completely covered in mould. Fixing the down pipe, putting a wardrobe heater in and using the dehumidifier helped, but this problem was not completely resolved until the piles were replaced.

When the piles were replaced we found that a new veranda had been built over the old wooden veranda which was now completely rotten; this was right outside our bedroom and our wardrobe; and this was the cause of the musty smell.

The DVS we installed, as with all similar systems circulates fresh air through the home even when we are away. The closed up house never smells stuffy and is much warmer and cosier now.

CHAPTER 7

Aristotle coined the phrase "the whole is greater than the sum of its parts". Meaning the complexities in the food we eat cannot replaced or copied without losing its completeness. Or That in its complete form it is perfect and greater than its individual parts.

"The Whole is Greater than the sum of its parts".

This phrase was coined by Aristotle one of the greatest philosophers of all time. Judged solely in terms of his philosophical influence, only Plato is his peer: Aristotle's works shaped centuries of philosophy from Late Antiquity through the Renaissance, and even today continue to be studied with keen, non-antiquarian interest.

A remarkable researcher and writer, Aristotle left a great body of work, perhaps numbering as many as two hundred treatises, from which approximately thirty-one survive.

His surviving writings span a wide range of disciplines, from logic, metaphysics and philosophy of mind, through ethics, political theory, aesthetics and rhetoric, and into such primarily non philosophical fields as empirical biology, where he excelled at detailed plant and animal observation and taxonomy.

The meaning of his words: ***"The Whole is Greater than the sum of its parts"*** are varied and can be applied in many situations.

In the plant world at least, can be explained when we look at an herb like Meadowsweet (Filipendula Ulmaria) for instance.

The herb is most useful in the gastrointestinal tract addressing a variety of problems including specifically **peptic ulceration**. Although the herb has aspirin like qualities another active constituent in the plant, **the mucilage**, protects the gut. Whereas the drug Aspirin(27) can cause artificially induced ulcers, water extracts of the whole herb have been found to protect against artificially induced ulcers including those caused by aspirin.

The conclusion therefore is that the aspirin like qualities in the herb Meadowsweet are accompanied with the gut protecting qualities of mucilage which are not in the drug Aspirin. A side effect of over using an anti- inflammatory drug like Aspirin could be the formation of stomach ulcers.

Why?

Because:

Aspirin is a man- made anti – inflammatory drug. Reducing inflammation is its one action. It has been manufactured for its ability to 1. Reduce inflammation, fever and pain. And

2. A blood thinning agent. By its specific action on one targeted enzyme in the body called cyclo-oxygenase, or COX.

Organic whole foods, in their original state with no tampering from man, is also greater than the sum of its parts. Nature's infinite wisdom still holds some mystery to us today. Even in these modern times we are still learning about plants. Some of the modern practices of cultivation and fertilization cannot compete with nature.

Especially when in draught, certified organic practices in land management recover much quicker than land fertilized with man-made chemicals.

The lush appearance of man- made and modified grasses do not hold the abundant root base of their organic partners and fail in draught where their natural partners flourish. More farmers in New Zealand today rely on nature's wisdom to let her magic work on livestock welfare. There is growing evidence that herbs, such as forage chicory and plantain can be high yielding and a beneficial source of highly palatable and nutritious feed for grazing livestock. Using species like this within a system can reduce reliance on concentrate feeds, especially for finishing which reduces production costs. Although chicory has been used in agriculture for some time, its use as a modern forage crop for livestock is relatively new. Much like chicory, plantain has only recently established itself as a viable forage crop for livestock production. Both chicory and plantain have large tap roots, which increases their tolerance to dry conditions, which may become increasingly important if climate variability continues.

"The Whole is Greater than the sum of its parts"

"Most people are willing to admit that the foundation of health is adequate nutrition. Few people, however, have studied the subject of nutrition sufficiently to recognize the fact that most of our ill health today is directly the result of malnutrition, by which we are actually starving to death among plentiful supplies of supposedly good foods."

Dr Royal Lee 1946. (28)

In 1941, Dr Royal Lee created the Lee Foundation for Nutritional Research that soon become the largest clearinghouse of such information in the world. The works of Dr Royal Lee, showed that vitamin deficiencies, due to processed foods, are responsible for most degenerative disease. From organic farming to food-based vitamins, from raw milk to fermented foods, Dr Lee set the course for the field of whole food nutrition.

"The Whole is Greater than the sum of its parts"

HIPPOCRATES was a Greek physician born in 460 BC on the island of Cos, Greece.

He became known as the founder of medicine and was regarded as the greatest physician of his time.

He based his medical practice on observations and on the study of the human body. He held the belief that illness had a physical and a rational explanation. He rejected the views of his time that considered illness to be caused by superstitions and by possession of evil spirits and disfavour of the gods.

Hippocrates held the belief that the body must be treated as a whole and not just a series of parts. He accurately described disease symptoms and was the first physician to accurately describe the symptoms of pneumonia, as well as epilepsy in children. He believed in the natural healing process of rest, a good diet, fresh air and cleanliness. He noted that there were individual differences in the severity of disease symptoms and that some individuals were better able to cope with their disease and illness than others. He was also the first physician that held the belief that thoughts, ideas, and feelings come from the brain and not the heart as others of his time believed.

Hippocrates travelled throughout Greece practicing his medicine. He founded a medical school on the island of Cos, Greece and began teaching his ideas. He soon developed an Oath of Medical Ethics for physicians to follow.

This Oath is taken by physicians today as they begin their medical practice. He died in 377 BC.

Today Hippocrates is known as the "Father of Medicine".

Hippocrates:

"Let food be your medicine and let medicine be your food"

Hippocrates was a great observer of health and wellbeing and he notes the need for rest, a good diet, fresh air and cleanliness. These are basic requirements to good health and all are completely in our hands. If we follow these simple rules we should be able to live a healthy life as long as we are disciplined.

In summing up, while we have made some advances in the nutritional value of whole foods compared to manufactured foods, we are still a long way from unlocking nature's secrets.

However I hope you are enlightened in the true value of the words

"The Whole is Greater than the sum of its parts"

And the importance of eating only fresh foods from the freshest sources available to you.

Other resources:

Heritage plants: *Visit: <u>Koanga Institute (29)</u>*

CHAPTER 8

The 1/3/ - 2/3 rule can be used as a simple guide to food portions.

1/3 - 2/3 Rule.

So far we have talked about: The number # 1 Rule for a long and healthy Life:

"Fresh is best forget the Rest"

Follow your unique Traditional Diet and why because "The Whole is greater than the sum of its Parts"

You now understand the importance of whole food and what whole food is. The importance of a traditional diet and why. Organic whole food grown without man-made fertilizers and pesticides, grown with natural plant allies that are sustainable, nutrient rich and do not harm the body. You understand the dangers of processed foods and how these foods have contributed to obesity, malnutrition and contamination of the food chain.

Now we will talk about the 1/3 - 2/3 rule.

In most cases the simplest rule to follow is 1/3 protein to 2/3 carbohydrates. When we talk of carbohydrates there are two groups low carbs are mostly fruit and vegetables that are low in starch. High carbs are sugars, a pure and refined carbohydrate with practically no fats, proteins, minerals or vitamins these foods should be avoided as they are regarded as naked carbohydrates meaning they have no nutritional value.

When the body consumes a naked carbohydrate, a food with no nutritional value, the body doesn't recognise it as a food. However to absorb and assimilate a naked carbohydrate the body can adjust by finding the nutrients from another source in the body which could be from any organ or bone.

Remember this quote from Dr Lee:

"Most people are willing to admit that the foundation of health is adequate nutrition. Few people, however, have studied the subject of nutrition sufficiently to recognize the fact that most of our ill health today is directly the result of malnutrition, by which we are actually starving to death among plentiful supplies of supposedly good foods."

Dr Lee 1946.

Processed Cereals:

Most ready- made packaged cereals are packed with sugar even if they say they are whole grain and healthy, the stuff athletes use.

Especially with any **puffed** grain, the process of producing the **puffed** effect as in: honey puffs, cocoa puffs, Nutri grain cereal and more, alters the structure of the grain, in a similar process to what is done to make margarine solid.

The grain is hydrogenated changing the molecular structure to create the puffed effect. And the process turns the food into a synthetic food that the body has no recognition of.

None of these manifested, man- made cereals can match the nutrient rich value of Whole Grain Oats. Choose Organic where possible and still save money on your grocery bill and gain a nutrient rich start to the day.

Dried Fruits: While dried fruits can be used in moderation it is important to note that dehydration increases the carbs count.

Low Fat Foods: The majority of low fat products and snacks have high carb levels to make them tasty. Check out labels before consuming.

Flours, cakes and biscuits: All high in carbs, white flour with virtually no nutrient value. If you are doing your own baking try spelt flour and notice the difference.

Each person is an individual and to work out portions needs some experimentation to figure out what makes you feel the best. I use my fist. And generally your fist size is a good guide for you.

For me it is best to eat a 1/3 portion of protein no bigger than my fist. The 2/3 of carbohydrates = 2 fists of low carbs or 1 fist low carbs + 1 fist high carbs. And 2 fists high carbs = 60 minutes vigorous exercise.

LOL

Your body will go through some adjustments when you make dietary changes. Some people may experience tiredness, headaches or just feel out of sorts or none of the above. In any case most of these symptoms will only last a short time no longer than a few weeks as your body detoxifies. Once your symptom free you will notice more energy, greater clarity, less tiredness, less allergies, less illness and an overall feeling of wellbeing as your body becomes nutrient rich and well nourished.

Note:

I think it is important to note how your body can deceive you into believing you actually need that bar of chocolate. I shouldn't pick on chocolate, because chocolate is wonderful after all, but I have heard people say I just need the chocolate to keep me going, my blood sugars are low, I'm feeling dizzy and chocolate will help. Stop right there! You've been tricked, mislead, swindled, double crossed, misinformed and duped by your own body. Have an apple instead.

Save the chocolate for those occasions when you can really indulge and enjoy without the hang-ups!

MY CHECKLIST FOR REDUCING COSTS

ENERGY

- *I turn off unused lights*
- *I use energy saver bulbs*
- *I switch off unused appliances, TV, computer, stereo, microwave and oven*
- *I dry clothes on the line and under veranda if wet*
- *I dress warmly rather than use the heater*
- *I installed a DVS system to reduce moisture and circulate fresh air in my home*
- *I have a dehumidifier to reduce moisture in my home*
- *I removed all damp areas from my home*

SHOPPING

- *I use canvas shopping bags*
- *I avoid pre- packed items where possible*
- *I buy locally*
- *I buy farm fresh free range eggs*
- *I buy meat from family with a lifestyle block*
- *I grow my own fruit and vegetables*
- *I support local grocers who buy local produce*
- *I don't buy things I can do without*
- *I recycle as much as I can*
- *I buy second hand*

WASTE

- *I recycle paper items – gift wrap, envelopes*
- *I recycle plastic containers*
- *I have a compost bin*
- *I donate used items to charity*
- *I print on both sides of paper*
- *I repair goods when they break, rather than just replacing them*

WATER

- *I have a front loader washing machine*
- *I use cold water washes and do only full loads*
- *I recycle washing machine water on my lawn*
- *I do not run the tap while brushing my teeth*
- *I use a half flush on the toilet*
- *I do not have dripping taps*
- *I insulated my hot water cylinder*
- *half fill the jug with cold water for a cuppa*
- *I have short showers and don't use the bath as much*
- *I hand wash dishes in a half full sink*

GENERAL

- *I use natural homemade non-toxic ingredients for cleaning*
- *I get bills emailed to me*
- *I patronize stores and organizations that have committed to environmental sustainability*
- *I walk to the shops*
- *Waste disposal is a cost to us all that we do not normally consider.*
- *These are hidden costs that one way or another we all pay for.*

However we can do small things in our daily lives that will make a major impact on our environment in a positive way and at the same time save a lot of money. Consider how we lived only 40 years ago, when we had no plastic bottles and no plastic shopping bags. Implementing these changes can save the planet and our finances.

CHAPTER 9

This chapter is all about growing food. Companion planting and preparing the soil.

In The Garden

I always wanted an outdoor water feature. A large ball with water tumbling over the edge in a recycling continuing flow. I would put it in the corner of the back yard where on a sunny day you can soak up the sun and listen to the sound of running water.

Bliss! ☺

That has never happened and I am over that now. I am satisfied with the sprinkler system I have installed myself covering all my vegetable, herb and flower-gardens.

My focus in recent times has been extending the vegetable garden to include potatoes, corn, kumara and more of the vegetables we eat.

That has never happened and I am over that now. I am satisfied with the sprinkler system I have installed myself covering all my vegetable, herb and flower-gardens. My focus in recent times has been extending the vegetable garden to include potatoes, corn, kumara and more of the vegetables we eat. If you have a bucket you can grow them. We even have dwarf varieties of fruit trees that can be grown in a large pot. Plants need water to carry nutrients and to soften the soil.

If you are growing in a bucket or pot try upending a bottle of water with a hole pierced in the lid to continuously drip-feed growing plants.

This is particularly useful if you cannot attend your plants for a few days. Simply refill the bottle when empty. Feed your plants with mulch, dry lawn clippings, old leaves, straw, hay, comfrey and dry manure.

Mulching will help to keep the weeds down and the soil moist.

You cannot overdo it.

HOME MADE LIQUID MANURE

Fill a bucket with weeds, nettles, comfrey, dried seaweed, chamomile or yarrow and cover with water. Put the lid on and leave for a week or two to brew. Use the liquid watered down by 50% as a liquid fertilizer for those plants that need a little extra help. Anything you have growing in a pot will require more feeding - once a fortnight will be ample. This combination is also good sprayed on your fruit trees to harden the wood in winter and strengthen the plants. Grow Comfrey as a border to your veggie garden - it will stop any grass from entering your garden.

Comfrey leaves also help break down plant matter in the compost bin.

(Comfrey is also useful in ointments and creams especially for broken bones).

Another herb Calendula which will grow all year round in the Waikato where I live. Calendula is a great companion herb which will help insulate vegetables from the colder days of winter.

Plant calendula in your vegetable garden to deter pests especially around your tomatoes - Calendula is a great companion plant. Plant your veggies in close proximity to help reduce weeds. Carrots are slow growers and require weeding, they do not need to be grown in nice long rows which give weeds a chance to prosper between each row; try planting carrots in bunches instead. Tight bunches of vegetables deter pests and is good for the soil - by the time they are half grown weeds will no longer be able to compete. Bare soil is more susceptible to wind and water damage as well as weeds which love to colonize in bare soil.

Planting nitrogen rich plants like peas, beans and sweet peas benefit the garden - as they decay mulch them back into the garden. Every time you pick something from your veggie crop try to plant something else in its place, even if it's mustard seed or radishes which can be turned back into the soil to enrich it for later planting.

Fruit trees as mentioned earlier can be grown in pots - they require more attention but will survive well. When shopping for your fruit trees you will find many new varieties of fruit that are perfect for container growing. Plant the fruit you like to eat and which will grow well in your area.

COMPANION PLANTING

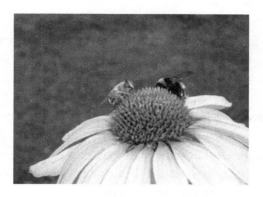

Companion planting combines vegetables that complement each other in the garden. They are a valuable asset in the living garden and this method of gardening has been practiced for centuries by different cultures. The Native American culture grew corn, beans and squash together, (known as the three sisters). The corn offers a structure for the beans to grow on; the beans offer the corn valuable nutrients, (corn are heavy feeders of nitrogen) and the squash offers ground cover to keep moisture in and stop the growth of weeds.

A living mulch for the three sisters to thrive together in harmony. Find a sunny spot in your garden and condition your soil ready for planting. Make a circular mound about a metre across at the highest point in the centre plant your corn – 9 seeds in a circle. Allow a 30cm space and plant your beans around your corn about 12 seeds.

Lastly plant your squash - 3 seeds either side of your circle.

Depending on how much corn, beans and squash you require this method can be repeated either in a long row or in a horse shoe shape. Corn and beans around the edge of the horse shoe and squash in the middle. As the squash grows it can spread out amongst the corn and beans. I found planting the corn first works better as the beans are vigorous growers.

When corn is 10cm high I plant the beans and Nasturtiums. I use nasturtiums because they are also high in nitrogen. Harmony in your garden can be achieved using these principles.

Different species of plants prefer to be together; they get along and the results speak for themselves on the dinner table. Companion planting recognises that some plants are beneficial to each other. By helping in their growth and wellbeing, as well as deter pests they also attract helpful insects like bees etc.

They will do this in many ways:

The smell of the volatile oils in the companion plant discourages certain pests.

Some plants have shapes which confuse the pest's recognition ability.

Some plants will attract beneficial insects like bees, which consequently pollinate them.

Some plants will attract insects which kill pests, or encourage birds to spread seeds etc.

Others simply enhance each other's growth by physical and energetic means. For instance tomatoes and marigolds love each other.

Plant basil, chilies and capsicum with your tomatoes.

The following list is a guide to use when planning your garden.

VEGETABLES

ALLIUMS: Onion, garlic, leek, shallot, chive

Allies: Fruit trees, tomato, pepper, potato, cabbage, broccoli and carrot.

Repel: slugs, aphids, Carrot fly and cabbage worm

Avoid: beans, peas, parsley

ASPARAGUS

Allies: Tomato, dill, coriander, parsley, basil, comfrey, marigold

Avoid: onion, garlic, potato

BRASSICA:

Broccoli, cabbage, Brussel-sprouts, cauliflower

Allies: geranium, dill, onion, shallot, garlic, rosemary, nasturtium,

Borage

Avoid: mustard, tomato, pepper, eggplant, chilli

BEANS: Good nitrogen fixer and fertilizer for some plants, too much for others

Allies: Corn, spinach, lettuce, rosemary, summer savory, dill, carrot, brassica, beet, radish, strawberry, cucumber

Avoid: Tomato, chilli, sunflower, onion, garlic, kale, cabbage, broccoli

BEETROOT:

Adds minerals to soil, 25% magnesium, (beans and beetroot stunt each other's growth)

Allies: lettuce, onion, catnip, garlic, brassica, mint

Avoid: beans

BROCCOLI

Allies: geranium, dill, rosemary, nasturtium, borage

Avoid: mustard, tomato, pepper

CABBAGE

Allies: geranium, dill, alliums, rosemary

Avoid: mustard, tomato, pepper, strawberry, beans

N.B. Rosemary repels cabbage flies; geraniums trap cabbage worms

CARROTS: Love nitrogen.

Tomatoes grow better with carrots but may stunt the carrots growth beans which are bad companions for tomatoes provide the nitrogen carrots need.

Allies: Tomato, alliums, lettuce, rosemary, wormwood, sage, beans

Avoid: dill, parsnip, radish

CELERY

Allies: cosmos, daisy, snapdragon

Avoid: corn

CORN

Allies: beans, sunflower, peas, cucumber, melons, parsley, potato,

Geranium

Avoid: tomato, celery

CUCUMBER

Allies: nasturtium, radish, marigold, sunflower, peas, beetroot, carrot, dill

Avoid: tomato, sage

EGGPLANT

Allies: beans, pepper, marigold, mint,

Avoid: runner beans

LEEKS

Allies: alliums, celery, apple trees, carrot

Repel: cabbage worms, aphids, carrot fly

Avoid: beans, peas

LETTUCE

Allies: radish, beans, carrot, mint including hyssop and sage

Repel: slugs

Avoid: celery, cabbage, cress, parsley

MUSTARDS

Allies: cabbage, cauliflower, radish, Brussel- sprouts and turnip

NIGHTSHADES:

tomato, eggplant, chilli, peppers, potato

Allies: carrot, alliums, oregano

Avoid: beans, black walnuts, corn, fennel, dill, brassica

PEPPERS

Allies: themselves, marjoram, tomato, geranium, petunia, basil

Avoid: beans, kale, cabbage, Brussel sprouts

Peppers like humidity, which can be helped by dense ground cover plants like marjoram (marjoram and oregano are the same plant), and basil; they also need direct sunlight.

The fruit can be harmed by sunlight therefore they grow well under tomatoes which can shelter the fruit and raise the humidity level - another example of three sisters.

ONIONS

Allies: tomato, kale, broccoli, cabbage alliums

Repel: aphids, carrot fly and other pests

Avoid: beans, peas, Leek

POTATOES

Allies: horseradish (increases disease resistance of potatoes)

Avoid: sunflowers, tomato

PUMPKIN / SQUASH

Allies: corn, beans, buckwheat, catnip, tansy, radish

Attract: spiders, ground beetles

SPINACH

Allies: beans, peas (natural shade)

TOMATOES

Allies: roses, pepper, basil, oregano, asparagus, parsley, carrot, marigold, alliums, celery, geranium, petunia, nasturtium, borage

Repel: asparagus beetle

Avoid: black walnut, corn, fennel, peas, dill, potato, beetroot, kale, rosemary.

HERBS

BASIL

Allies: tomato, pepper, oregano, asparagus, petunia, chamomile, anise

Repel: asparagus beetle, mosquito, flies

Avoid: rue, sage

Chamomile and anise increase basil's essential oils and make tomatoes taste better.

BORAGE

Allies: almost everything, especially strawberries, cucumber, tomato and gourds

Attracts: predatory insects, honeybee

Repel: many pests **Borage is the magic bullet of companion plants**

CARAWAY

Allies: strawberries

Attracts: parasitic wasps, parasitic flies

CHAMOMILE

Allies: basil, wheat, onion, cabbage, cucumber (growing near other herbs increases their essential oils which repel pests

Attracts: hoverflies, wasps

CHERVIL:

Loves shade; grow beside shade tolerant plants; will make radishes spicier

Allies: lettuce, radish, broccoli

Repel: aphids

CORIANDER

Allies: spinach, beans, peas

Repel: aphids

CHIVES

Allies: apples, carrot, tomato, brassica, many others

Repel: cabbage worms, carrot fly, aphids

Avoid: beans, peas

Same companion traits as all alliums are said to prevent apple scab after 3 years planting at the base of your apple trees

DILL:

One of the few plants said to grow with fennel Allies: cabbage, corn, lettuce, onion, cucumber

Attracts: hoverflies, wasps, tomato horn worms, honey bees

Repel: aphids, spider mites, squash bugs

Avoid: carrot, tomato

FENNEL

Allies: dill

Attracts: ladybugs

Repel: aphids

Avoid: almost anything

Fennel can actually kill many garden plants; however by attracting lady bugs they are worth their weight in gold, as lady bugs eat many garden pests including white fly.

GARLIC

Allies: apple trees, pear trees, roses, cucumber, peas, lettuce, celery

Repel: aphids, cabbage looper, ants, rabbits, cabbage maggot

HYSSOP:

Stimulates the growth of grapes

Allies: cabbage, grapes

Attract: honeybees, butterflies

Repel: cabbage moth larvae, cabbage butterflies

LOVAGE:

Like borage and geraniums another magic bullet

Allies: beans, almost all plants

Attracts: wasps, ground beetles

Avoid: rhubarb

OREGANO

Allies: tomato, pepper, many other plants

Repel: aphids

Ground cover and humidity for pepper plants if allowed to spread among them

PEPPERMINT

Allies: all brassica

Repel: cabbage fly

ROSEMARY

Allies: sage, cabbage, beans, carrot

Repel: bean beetle, bean parasites

SAGE

Allies: rosemary, cabbage, beans, carrot

Attracts: honey bees

Repel: cabbage fly, carrot fly, black flea beetle, cabbage looper, cabbage maggot, many bean parasites

SOUTHERNWOOD

Allies: fruit trees

Repel: controls cabbage moths and mosquito

SPEARMINT

Repel: aphids, ants

SUMMER SAVORY

Allies: green beans, onion

TANSY

Allies: beans, cucumber, squash, corn, roses etc.

Attract: honey bees

Repel: flying insects, Japanese beetle, striped cucumber beetle, squash bugs, ants

Generally repels all insects except the nectar eating variety.

FLOWERS

GERANIUM

Allies: roses, tomato, pepper, grape

Repel: leafhopper, Japanese beetle

A trap crop that attracts pests away from roses and grape vines; Attracts leaf hoppers, carrier of the curly top virus, away from tomatoes, peppers, eggplant

MARIGOLD

Allies: most plants, especially tomato, pepper, cucumber, gourd, brassica

Repel: other pests

Marigolds are a wonder drug for the companion plant world invoking the saying, 'Plant them everywhere in your garden'. French marigolds produce a pesticide from their roots so strong that it lasts years after they have gone.

PETUNIA

Allies: asparagus, cucumber, pumpkin

Repel: leaf hopper, Japanese beetle, aphid, asparagus beetle

Almost identical to geraniums - a trap crop

NASTURTIUM

Allies: many plants, melon, cucumber, gourd, beans, tomato, apple trees, brassica

Attract: predatory insects

Repel: aphid, cabbage looper, squash bug, white fly, cucumber beetle

Avoid: cauliflower, radish

Best plant to attract predatory insects.

SUNFLOWER

Allies: corn, tomato

Repel: aphid; ants herd aphids into sunflower plants keeping them away from other neighbouring plants

TANSY

Allies: cucumber, squash, raspberry and relatives, roses, corn

Attract: sugar ants, Japanese beetle, cucumber beetle, squash, bugs and mice

Toxic to many animals - do not plant where stock graze

YARROW

Allies: many plants

Attract: predatory wasps, lady bugs, hover-flies

Improves soil quality and enriches the compost heap

ALFALFA:

Improves the soil, fixes nitrogen like beans do, breaks up hard soil, attracts lady bugs and parasitic wasps

Trees

APPLE

Allies: clover, chives, garlic, leek, nasturtium, southernwood

WALNUT

Black walnut is harmful to the growth of all nightshade plants: tomato, pepper, eggplant, potato, paprika, chilli, petunia etc.

CHAPTER 10

Why a healthy diet and saving the planet are the same thing.

How good would it be to feel GREAT for the rest of your life better than you have felt in years? What's it worth to you?

In 1988 we reached a population of 5 billion people in the world.

We reached a tipping point where the earths ability to repair the damage man had made was lost and the damage man made to the planet took over.

The environmental pollutants from the industrial revolution in the early 1800 to the agricultural chemical revolution of post WW2 – have accumulated and persisted in our environment to such a level it is now causing damage and chronic disease to accelerate.

With the production of fertilizers, pesticides, herbicides, PCBs DDTs, phthalates and <u>83000 other chemicals (30)</u> released into our environment human health and the survival of our planet is under threat.

For as long as man has existed the body's number one defence system against disease has been the immune system. With good nutrition the immune system is able to deal with parasites, molds, bacteria, fungus, viruses and bugs.

And although the body can deal with and expel many harmful chemicals the added burden on the immune system has been overwhelming for a growing number of people who suffer chronic disease.

Now in today's world more of us are suffering and living with some form of chronic disease.

<u>For the first time in history life expectancy is falling.(31)</u>

Now is the time to STOP our bad habits and change our ways, or life as we know it will no longer exist. We can all do our bit to help. The way to start is to nurture yourself and do nothing to harm mother-nature anymore.

We Must Become Organic to Survive.

We have to reduce our dependence on these chemicals and revert back to nature to allow mother earth time to rejuvenate and put the balance back in our favour before we can eliminate our burden of poor health.

The food we eat has the power to unburden our immune system and restore wellbeing. Food is information that has the power to CURE chronic disease.

Food has the power to CURE FLC (feeling like crap)

And according to Dr Naviaux:

"I believe that the rules of acute care medicine rely on the body's natural healing pathways to remain intact. This requirement does not hold for chronic disease. In chronic disease, the normal healing cycle is blocked, so full recovery, when treated with current medicines almost never happens".

Dr Robert Naviaux(32) *MD, PhD is Professor of Medicine, Paediatrics, and Pathology at the University of California, San Diego (UCSD) School of Medicine. He is the founder and co-director of the Mitochondrial and Metabolic Disease Centre and former President of the Mitochondrial Medicine Society (MMS).*

There is no drug on the planet that has the power to change your health so dramatically, every bite of food is information and if you put junk in you get junk out.

It's so easy! Leave the food that man made and eat the food that mother-nature made.

"Organic"

The word organic was invented by the food industry because if they called their food herbicide, pesticide, preservative, artificial colouring and artificial flavouring food.

I don't think we would buy it.

Eat food with no bar code. An avocado has no bar code.

Eat local food – because local food has the power to resist all the toxins of your local environment. They have managed to grow and thrive in the very environment we live in therefore those foods will pass on to you the protection it created to grow.

I say: Eat to Beat Disease and Save the Planet.

Food helps – The first line of defence – heal the gut and heal the disease – prebiotics and Probiotics – creating a healthy gut and bacterial environment. Activated charcoal and fulvic acid assist in moving heavy metals and other toxins from the body.

In short become your own doctor. Learn to help you and your loved ones with day to day problems. Get your life back so you can do the things that matter.

Reprogram your body, choose foods that nourish you and access food differently.

Before you take the first bite say to yourself is this good for my body and my planet?

It doesn't take long either, just 7 days of good food can reverse 15 years of suffering bad health.

Jan was overweight, had high cholesterol, congestive heart failure and pre diabetic – she lost almost 20 kilo's and was off all her meds in 3 months. This is unheard of in main stream medicine. You get your meds and you stay on them for life? And often require more meds to counter the side effects of the other meds you are on.

Can you see where this is going eh!

Imagine if you had a million dollar race horse?

Would you feed it junk food?

Only if you were an idiot right!

You have this amazing investment – would you hurt it-

But aren't you worth it – of course you are – you are worth a whole lot more – so why would you hurt yourself and put junk in your one and only beautiful body.

I don't want to deprive myself, but if you're eating bad food aren't you really depriving yourself of what you really want the most which is your good health and energy?

Being sick is expensive. I want to invite you to rethink health. Food matters, health is 80% diet, 20% is everything else.

Move more. You don't have to go out and run a marathon just move more in your day. Park the car further away so you have a longer walk to your destination. Do 10 squats before you eat, more movement is building resilience.

Just remember this: bacteria grows in a stagnant pond.

Your lymphatic system (is stagnant and requires us to move to activate it) in the body removes waste, dead cells and debris. It requires movement to help eliminate waste from the body. All I ask is for you to move **often**.

Heal yourself first. Then think about serious exercise.

Thoughts matter too.

The Rules of the Mind.

- Every thought you think causes a physical reaction and an emotional response within you.
- What is expected tends to be realised.
- In a battle with emotion and logic, emotion always wins.
- Your mind always does what you think it will do.
- Your mind works to move you from pain to pleasure
- Your mind responds to the pictures and words you install
- The mind learns by repetition
- The mind cannot hold conflicting beliefs or thoughts they cancel each other out.
- Your mind does not care if what you say is good, bad, true, false, healthy, unhealthy, right or wrong. It acts on your words regardless

"DIRT FOOD BACTERIA AND HUMAN HEALTH

We are seeing an ever-increasing burden of chronic disease, primarily driven by our food and food system. This is perpetuated by agricultural, food and health care policies that don't support health. We need to rethink disease and reimagine a food system and a health care system that protects health, unburdens the economy from the weight of obesity and chronic disease, protects the environment, help reverse climate change and create a nation of healthy children and citizens". Dr Mark Hyman. MD (33)

My sentiments too.

Let's sum up:

The Number # 1 Rule for Living a Long and Healthy Life.

If there was only 1 rule you had to follow for Living a Long and Healthy Life. Would you do it?

YES – it's easy –"Fresh is Best Forget the Rest".

If you are suffering from an allergy or illness and you follow this 1 rule you will reduce Your Symptoms and reverse Your Dis-ease altogether.

YES – I now avoid the foods that could cause my allergies, inflammation or illness.

What if I said if you follow this 1 rule you will Lose Weight and keep it off forever?

YES – Because I only eat fresh food now and I have eliminated eating hidden sugars found in processed foods from my diet.

How about if I said by following this 1 rule you could also Save Money. Would you do it?

YES – Because I am no longer paying for the processing, packaging and preparation of the food I now eat.

And if I said by following this 1 rule you could support Local Industry and Local Jobs.

YES – Because what I buy now is local fresh produce.

By following this 1 rule you can also Reduce Household Waste.

YES – by eating fresh foods I no longer have to deal with all the pre-packaging that comes with processed foods.

Follow this 1 rule and you will be helping to Save Your Planet.

YES – because I have reduced waste, eliminated synthetic food and all the packaging that comes with it.

And what if I said if you follow this 1 rule you may never have to visit your doctor or never have to worry about medical bills again and provide a better future for our children.

Yes – because I no longer eat the foods that have caused my health issues. And with the information I have now I can ensure my children are aware of the benefits of eating fresh. "

"Fresh is Best Forget the Rest".

You're Bonus Material

1/ 10 Essential foods to optimize brain function

By Deborah Harper from: www.happyhomesnz.com

To increase your chances of healthy, optimized brain function select the best fuel possible. Elevate your mood, enthusiasm, drive, pleasure and clarity.

Specific **"smart"** foods can easily be included in your daily diet to improve brain function and to slow the aging process. Avoid those foods that clog, fog and age the brain. Foods to avoid include processed fast foods and sugary fatty foods. When consuming processed fast foods the body is burdened by extra work.

White sugar is a naked carbohydrate stripped of all goodness, to process this type of sugar the body has to make up the shortfall in nutrients which it steals from you. White processed sugar also found in so called energy drinks can give you the instant high- energy boost you are looking for but this is short lived and can leave you feeling tired, sad, irritated and anxious. Specific foods in nature's bounty fuel your brain for optimum performance and actually make you smarter.

1 Eat more fish

(EFAs) Essential fatty acids high in Omega 3's are found in oily fish including salmon, trout, mackerel, herring, sardines, pilchards and kippers.

Also found in linseed (flaxseed) oil, soya bean oil, pumpkin seeds, walnut oil and soya beans.

Lasting powers of concentration and the continuous flow of oxygen from blood sugars to feed brain cells are paramount.

EFAs are essential for good brain function helping to protect the myelin sheath which is the insulation surrounding nerve fibres enabling the free flow of messages throughout the brain.

2 Are you getting your Oats?

Organic whole grains – oats, whole-grain breads, and brown rice can reduce the risk for heart disease and will lift your mood, high in fibre B vitamins and slow releasing sugars whole-grains can keep you buoyant all day.

Information is carried between the cells in the brain by chemicals called neurotransmitters - and these play a key role in your mood.

One of the key neurotransmitters is dopamine, the 'feel - good' messenger.

High levels of dopamine give you enthusiasm, drive and pleasure. Falling levels make you feel sad, empty, bored and irritated. I like to call it "the give me give me more hormone".

Fatty sugary foods might give you that instant energy and gratification with a surge of dopamine, however this is short lived. Whereas slow release – protein rich foods like "porridge for breakfast will keep you going all day".

Other foods such as beets, eggs, almonds, meat and soybeans include important molecules used to manufacture dopamine.

Bacon and eggs for breakfast will also keep you going all day because of tryptophan which the brain uses to manufacture serotonin responsible for contentment and reducing anxiety. I like to think of serotonin as the "I'm happy I don't need anything else hormone".

3 Broccoli is Brain food

Broccoli is high in vitamin K, which is known to enhance cognitive function and improve brainpower.

Dark green leafy vegetables, fish, liver, kelp, soybeans, egg yolks, alfalfa, yoghurt, strawberries, peas, carrots, cauliflower, papaya, safflower and more all contain vitamin K which is also responsible for vitality and longevity. In healthy people vitamin K is produced in the gastrointestinal tract by specific bacteria, a healthy stomach is an important factor in full nutrient absorption.

4 Fruit & Veg

Fruit and vegetables have almost all the vitamins amino acids and minerals humans need to survive well and healthy. Vitamin C present in most fresh fruit and vegetables has long been thought to have the power to increase mental agility. Acting as an antioxidant protecting other vitamins and body tissue from injury, pollution, poisons and free radicals. While also helping to maintain the strength of blood vessel walls particularly those of tiny capillaries and one of the best sources of this vital vitamin is blackcurrants. High in vitamin C they pack 218 times the recommended daily dose per serving. Loaded with antioxidants they are a major boost for the immune system.

5 Tomatoes

Tomatoes - *Lycopene* is a carotenoid and phytonutrient found in red fruits and vegetables such as tomatoes, pink grapefruits, watermelons and papayas.

It is the compound that is responsible for the red colour in these foods. There is good evidence to suggest that lycopene, a powerful antioxidant could help protect against the kind of free radical damage to cells which occurs in the development of <u>dementia, particularly Alzheimer's. (34)</u>

Lycopene may help prevent DNA damage in the cells and help the cells to function better.

High levels of lycopene, in the blood and fatty tissues, correlate with reduced risk of cancer, heart disease and macular degeneration.

6 Blueberries you bet

Blueberries - a regular diet with fresh blueberries in season improves your memory.

Blueberries are a major source of flavonoids, in particular anthocyanins and flavanols.

Although the precise mechanisms by which these plant-derived molecules affect the brain are unknown, they have been shown to cross the blood brain barrier after dietary intake.

It is believed that they exert their effects on learning and memory by enhancing existing neuronal (brain cell) connections, improving cellular communications and stimulating neuronal regeneration.

The enhancement of both short-term and long-term memory is controlled at the molecular level in neurons.

Recent research was able to show that the ability of flavonoids to enhance memory are mediated by the activation of signalling proteins via a specific pathway in the hippocampus, the part of the brain that controls learning and memory.

7 Vital Vitamins

Brewer's yeast

B vitamins – found in green leafy vegetables, broccoli, legumes, liver, kidney, orange juice, brewer's yeast and more is necessary for the formation of red blood cells and is a part of every gene and chromosome in every cell.

Concentrated in spinal and extracellular fluid it is essential for mental and emotional health stress and fatigue.

B6, B12 and folic acid - are known to reduce levels of homocysteine in the blood.

Elevated levels of homocysteine are associated with increased risk of stroke, cognitive impairment and Alzheimer's disease.

High doses of B6, B12 and folic acid can significantly reduce brain shrinkage.

8 Able Avocado

Avocados are almost as good as blueberries in promoting brain health while avocado is a fatty fruit, it is important to note it is a monounsaturated fat, which contributes to healthy blood flow.

"And healthy blood flow means a healthy brain,"

9 Go Nuts

Avocados also lower blood pressure, high blood pressure is a risk factor for the decline in cognitive abilities, a lower blood pressure should promote brain health.

Avocados are high in calories, just adding just 1/4 to 1/2 of an avocado to one daily meal as a side dish is all you need.

Nuts and seeds. Nuts and seeds are good sources of vitamin E and higher levels of vitamin E correspond with less cognitive decline as you get older.

Responsible for protecting vitamins A and C and increases the ability of white blood cells to resist infection.

Found in walnuts, hazelnuts, brazil nuts, almonds, cashews, peanuts, sunflower seeds, sesame seeds, flax seed, or organic un-hydrogenated nut butters such as peanut butter, almond butter, and tahini.

Raw or roasted doesn't matter, although if you're on a sodium restricted diet, try unsalted nuts.

When consumed daily they are very satisfying and make a great alternative to snacking on comfort food.

10 Herbs

I will just briefly mention a few herbs here Withania Somnifera, Gotu Kola, Ginkgo Biloba and many more I recommend you take with professional advice.

However Sage, Garlic, Ginger and Rosemary are easily available foods you can use liberally.

Rosemary tea is particularly uplifting make sure to drink this during the day only if you want to sleep at night.

A brain enhancing herbal tea can be made with 3 sage leaves, 3 thin slices of ginger and a small spring of rosemary in a cup pour over boiling water and infuse 3 minutes.

Strain, discard the herb and drink hot or cold sweeten with a little honey if desired.

2/ How to Gain More by Spending Less

I am old enough to remember groceries in boxes and paper shopping bags, the local green grocer, butcher and baker.

We had crates of beer, flagons and cardboard packed cans. It was common to have preserves, bottling fruit, pickles and chutney, freezing garden harvests of beans, carrots, corn, broccoli and cauliflower.

Mending clothes, knitting, dress making, curtain making and darning socks. Water came from taps.

When water in plastic bottles was first introduced I thought, this will never catch on, fancy buying Water, I will never buy water – it is just plain stupid.

Yeah right! I have since bought water, the plastic bottle is handy to carry around refill and use a few times before disposing of.

Now you can make plastic from air! Yes! Plastic can be made by sucking CO2 from the air. A US company called Newlight Technologies.

We had homemade tomato sauce - have you ever tasted it? Pure gold, nothing like the product you buy on the supermarket shelf. Delicious home grown tomatoes, onions, apples, vinegar and a few spices; that's all, nothing else.

I was talking to a friend the other day who was boasting about the home made tomato sauce her husband had been given for Christmas from a colleague at work.

His colleague's partner, had made it quite clear in a menacing tone, "You're bloody lucky to be getting that, because I wouldn't share it". The comment made him want to hide it and protect his precious gift from view.

Home grown food is delicious, fresh and full of premium wholesome, healthy nutrients. You know what has gone into producing home grown and the cost is minimal to you and to the environment.

No transport miles, no loss in nutrient value, no *(oil based)* plastic bags or packaging to carry it home, no unknown sprays, fertilizers or chemicals. Just pure and fresh premium home grown.

This was highlighted recently with my home grown tomatoes. I have a great spot that grows fantastic tomatoes up against the shed. They grow so well there and produce masses every year in the same place. Although it is recommended you change the places to grow tomatoes every year, it just didn't work for me.

Friends of ours had just come back from living overseas for a few years and we gave them some tomatoes to take home. Next time we saw them they raved about them, what flavour! So tasty! So delicious!

We have all been disappointed buying fruit or vegetables and they have looked so much better than they taste. The benefit of home grown fruit and vegetables is worth the effort and as it turns out is also a huge benefit to our health.

If you haven't got any garden space you would be surprised just what can be grown in a bucket or vertical garden. Growing our own fruit, vegetables and herbs can not only feed us they can be excellent household cleaners, air fresheners, pest repellents and home remedies.

Fruit trees can be as espaliers which takes much less space.

Who would have thought that this will not only improve your prosperity it will also improve your health. So just like granny, we can get out the spade, the preserving jars, jam pot and seeds, pull up our sleeves and get on with the job.

It's about taking control of your health, doing it for yourself and your family.

Recent history has proven that the world as we know it can change in a snap of the fingers we are slowly recovering from a recession. New Zealand endured the recession along with the rest of the world, but recovered quicker than most and today in 2014 we have all but recovered.

But it highlighted a point to me. I can live on less and reduce waste by making a few changes in the way I do things. I do not have to be the type of consumer I was pre-recession. It was something that had never really occurred to me until the global recession. Large corporations fell over around us like a domino effect, greed was the cause, even when some of those companies were helped by their governments they still failed.

But who would believe that with less spending our health will improve.

It happened in WW2 with "food rationing" - could this be the answer to our overloaded health system?

Just simply eating home grown produce?

Limited availability of basics like butter, flour, eggs and milk required more reliance on what we could get from our home garden.

What you put in is what you get out, and many of the diseases that clog our hospitals today are simply symptoms of a bad diet.

We can include conditions in this list such as:

Acne, Arthritis, Chronic fatigue, Colic, Constipation, Gastric Ulcers, Diabetes, Heart disease, Obesity, Crohn's disease, Irritable Bowel syndrome, Cancer, Asthma, Hay fever, Eczema, - the list goes on ...

I have worked in the health industry, in a public hospital, in regional referrals and in emergency. When working in that environment you get to see just how many people turn up there with serious eating/food related dis-ease.

I am also a Natural Medicine Practitioner, (a Medical Herbalist), I would have to say the majority of clients who came to see me had already tried conventional medicine which failed to solve their problem or the cure was worse than the disease.

In my experience I would put herbal medicine at the top of my list when comparing it to conventional medicine, for its ability to remedy so many of the above mentioned ailments especially any digestive problem.

The biggest difference being that conventional medicine treats the symptoms which masks the condition, while the body repairs itself. Whereas herbal medicine treats the underlying cause, by improving the entire digestive process.

Exercise is very important as well and 30 minutes brisk walking daily is probably the most beneficial exercise one can take up - **it's free** - 30 minutes time out for yourself and 30 minutes of fresh air daily. It is kind to your joints and is an excellent weight bearing exercise.

Simple fresh home grown food was normal when I was a child and in New Zealand today many primary schools have a vegetable garden where children learn to grow vegetables.

They are developing a skill that our grandparents knew about with the advantage of knowing that by doing so they will ensure a healthier future nutritionally. And the children love it. They are always enthusiastic in the garden. Gardening has really caught on.

3/ Detox Me Completely and Safely

Just browsing through the internet will show you that detox diets are big business. I have a college that regularly detoxes with some new liquid concoction that is going to work miracles. But the truth is she is just making her body go into survival mode until she eats normally again.

The cold truth is that you could be doing more harm than good.

Mary E. Pritchard, Ph.D. summed it up this way,

"The only thing I've ever seen yo-yo dieting do is lead to weight gain and self-doubt."

And from Michelle May Author of the Eat what you love and love what you eat series of books.

"Mindful eating requires awareness, intention, trust, new skills, practice – and revolutionary thinking".

Now is the time for a new revolution!

I call it, ***"Detox Me Completely and Safely".***

I'm not really one for fad diets and all the emotional coercion that comes from following them.

But as you know I am an advocate for healthy food and healthy eating. I believe certain foods to be medicine for certain health conditions. Did you know that 2 cups of strong black coffee can reduce the symptoms of an asthma attack.

And that avoiding dairy could reduce or even cure asthma symptoms due to undiagnosed intolerance?

I have never seen a detox diet that also considers the environment you live in? By that I mean rather than our internal environment, there are plenty of small things we can do to improve our surroundings and at the same time reduce our exposure to toxins.

Let's start in the home.

Household cleaners are full of <u>toxins (35)</u> that could have an adverse effect on your wellbeing. And one story that comes to mind is Beth Greer's

Beth was diagnosed with a herniated disk that turned out to be a golf ball sized tumour in her chest. Three surgeons agreed it needed to be removed. But this was in an area of the body packed with nerves and presented a very risky surgery. Beth weighed up her options and decided to avoid surgery to see if there wasn't something she could do for herself. Beth had always followed a good diet and exercise regularly. There was nothing more she could do there, so it had to be something else. She decided she would find out everything she could about her condition and found that tumours grow in response to irritation and inflammation. Therefore environmental toxins might be contributing to her tumours growth. This seemed like a practical first step. She went through her cupboards and threw out all the household cleaners and started from scratch making her own. And Beth cured her tumour. By throwing out all the products Beth had been using and replacing them with natural home made products.

Beth found her tumour reduced in size and disappeared completely in just 9 months.

I also remember the story of a student in nutrition classes who had an awful rash all over her face. She asked her tutor for some help because she didn't know what could be causing it. The tutor went through everything in her diet and found the culprit which was all the vitamin supplements she was taking.

On her tutors advice she immediately stopped taking the supplements to see what happen. A week or two later the rash was completely gone.

Your skin is the largest organ in your body and one of its roles is to eliminate toxins via the sweat glands. Her body was merely rejecting what it saw as waste.

Another product we all use that could be harmful is antiperspirant. I have seen sensational headlines on the internet claiming: "The leading cause of breast cancer (36) is the use of antiperspirant". Yes,

"ANTIPERSPIRANT"

The lymph glands in the armpits is where the problem occurs. And an antiperspirant is designed to stop perspiration. Which in turn stops the elimination of toxins from your body. Try a deodorant instead or best of all a crystal rock deodorant (37).

Another product we use often is Shampoo (38)

Or how about <u>hair dyes (39)</u>

Both of which have been associated with numerous forms of cancer but do not fear there are plenty of natural and safe alternatives out there too.

The point is, should you feel the need for a good detox, before you delve into the latest detox diet, have a thought for what else you can do to detox YOU.

And at the same time do the whole family a favour.

Open up your cupboards and read the labels on all the household cleaners, shampoos, hair dyes, cosmetics and antiperspirants. And if they are full of toxins get rid of them, replace them with safe natural alternatives. I'm sure you will notice the difference in no time at all.

The Ultimate Detox Diet

Finally, the best natural detox for everyone is to follow is a diet of fresh food grown in your area. Remember "fresh is best forget the rest" and eat the food that is "in season" which means in winter eat mainly root vegetables that grow at that time of year and in summer eat plenty of fresh fruit and vegetables that grow at that time of year.

Also try to eat a traditional diet from your country of origin. I don't mean don't eat anything foreign. That's fine to do so now and again. But if you eat a diet that is familiar to you and your origins then you are less likely to have an adverse effect.

Eat three times daily and the main meal of the day should include portions on your plate which consist of 2/3 fruit and vegetables and 1/3 meat/protein. The portion of meat/protein should be no bigger than your own fist. Drink plenty of fluids and exercise daily, a 30 minute brisk walk in the fresh air is best.

Lastly the liver is the great body cleanser and the best food for the liver is anything bitter. Bitter foods stimulate digestion and a good functioning liver is what will detox YOU.

The liver has a number of functions, but its main role in the digestive system is the processing of nutrients that are absorbed from the small intestine. Bile from the liver released into the small intestine also plays a crucial role in digesting fat.

Common Bitter Foods:

Chicory, Chard, Endive, Artichokes, Cress, Broccoli, Cabbage, Brussel Sprouts, Lettuce, Dandelion, Rocket, Cucumbers, Pumpkin, Melons, Mushrooms, Lemon juice, Grape fruit juice, Beer, Wine, Coffee and more....

4/ *My Little Pot of Gold*

For many years now I have used Calendula ointment for a huge range of ailments: Bites, scratches, sores, eczema, nappy rash, cradle cap and pretty much almost every minor injury you can think of. My children use it and now my grandchildren.

I sold it in my shop, online and I have even taught school children how to grow the plant, dry the flowers and make the ointment.

Now I want to share it with you.

Some things are so precious they must be shared and my "Little Pot of Gold" will be one of the most useful ointments you will have in your first aid cabinet. I am a Medical Herbalist taught in the art of traditional medicine. When I graduated I opened my shop in town which was a fantastic little business where I was happy for many years.

One of my best products was Calendula ointment, which is very easy to make. It makes fantastic gifts for friends and family but most of all it is extremely satisfying to create such a beneficial ointment.

This herb is known as the "weather forecaster" - if the petals are still closed at 7 am then it will rain.

The herbal marigold is the single variety with 2-3 flat rows of petals surrounding a brownish circular centre. The branching stem and oval leaves are pale green, slightly hairy and sticky to touch, with a strong odour. The tap-root is white and fleshy. The seeds of Calendula cover all possibilities. The outer seeds being crescent-shaped burrs (good for latching on to passing animals or humans) a circle of crescent moon shaped seeds and circular ones in the centre.

Calendula is an annual.

Easy to grow from seed with a 4-14 day germination period but once established will readily self-seed. I planted two Calendula plants a couple of years ago and now I have hundreds. Happy to grow all year round Calendula is frost resistant and enjoys a sunny situation and good garden soil.

This is a plant that enjoys harvesting.

Nipping the flower heads off encourages the plant to bush up and flower even more profusely.

Who would have thought using this herb in your daily diet would be of benefit to your health?

Parts used: Flower heads, the leaves can be used but are not very effective.

Internally Calendula is beneficial for stomach and duodenal ulcers. Known as a **liver tonic** it has an antiseptic effect on the liver and gallbladder, viral infections of the liver, other liver disorders, artery and capillary haemorrhage and also effective in delaying menstruation and normalizing the menstrual cycle.

It is a must in body lotions especially if you have varicose veins.

Externally calendula is an excellent herb for skin problems:

Inflammation, infection, bruising, cuts, ulcers, slow healing wounds, minor burns, oily skin, scalds, warts and eczema.

DRYING CALENDULA PETALS

To dry Calendula flowers it is best to collect them after it has rained once the petals have dried in the sun. Always collect herbs once all moisture from dew and rain has gone. Collect the full flower head by nipping it with your fingers just under the base. Place them evenly without touching on a tray and store in a dry airing cupboard. While it's hot and sunny I might leave them in the sun for the day, then move them to my hot water cupboard.

They will take 2-3 days to completely dry out.

If you have a dehydrator, place on trays as above then put dehydrator on low for 2 hours and then medium for 2 hours. When the flower heads are completely dry put in a brown paper bag and store in a dark dry place.

Calendula is unique among herbs, you will find this herb loses its colour fast in just 3-4 weeks. While this does not affect the quality of the herb, this is the best time to make your oil because the ointment will have a more intense colour.

The dried flowers will still be effective for 6 months or more but the ointment will not be as vibrant looking.

"MY LITTLE POT OF GOLD"

Every home should have calendula ointment in the medicine cabinet for day to day first aid. Use for babies' skin conditions and nappy rash, all wounds and inflamed lesions, boils, chilblains, fungal infection, bruises, eczema, acne **and the best lip balm ever.**

To make an oil lotion or ointment, pack the freshly dried flower heads into a sterilized jar and cover with oil.

I generally use olive oil, however other good quality oils can be used. Seal and label the jar with the name of the herb, the date you made it and count six weeks for the date that it will be ready to process.

Note: 2-6 weeks is fine.

Then place the jar in a sunny spot. This herb seems to soak up sun rays and just loves a sunny position. Generally I put it someplace where I will see it every day and remember to shake the bottle.

It is important not to allow any of the plant material to dry out.

After six weeks your herb is ready to use as an oil, great to add to babies bath, use as a massage oil, a base for your favourite dressings for salads, or to make into an ointment.

How to make Ointment

Drain oil into a pot squeezing excess through a sieve. The remaining plant material may be added to your compost heap.

Add beeswax to the oil (which may be bought from a chemist or the best beeswax is from a local honey maker) and place on very low heat to melt the beeswax slowly. This also helps to reduce damaging the oil.

Pour into a sterilized jar and cool. At this point I often add essential oil for extra aromatherapy. For children I recommend Lavender or Chamomile and for me Rose Otto, my favourite.

I use about **2 parts oil to 1 part beeswax._**

When it has cooled and solid, if your ointment is too hard, reheat and add a little more oil. If not hard enough, reheat and add a little more beeswax.

In this medium your ointment will last for many years.

Nothing is ever as good as your own handmade ointment made with **love.**

Feel free to pass this recipe on to all your friends and family. It is hard to believe that something so simple, grown in your own garden and made by you could so remarkably effective. I have customers who cannot believe the results.

"So fast, amazing how it stops the itch immediately. It works better than any eczema ointment I have ever used".

"Awesome for new tattoos, the new tattoo doesn't even crust up".

"Best lip balm I've ever used".

"Works wonders on my varicose veins".

"Remarkable how quickly it cleared up my infection".

TIP:

I've used Vicks Vapour Rub for years for colds. Try a blend of the two to accelerate recovery.

Rub calendula ointment on baby's feet, then use Vicks over top. The calendula ointment will stop the burning sensation of Vicks.

Try it and you'll see, just one thing, please let me know how it worked for you, I would **Love your feedback.**

ABOUT THE AUTHOR

What impact will I make in my life? I guess that will occur to all of us at some time in our life. My sister died of cancer when she was only 39. I have always thought life is short, she was so beautiful, the best sister anyone could have, my best friend. So how can I add real value in my life, what do I know that I can share with people that will allow them to have the best life possible? I have worked in the health industry, a health food shop, a medical centre and hospital. All experiences highlighted one thing to me: **"Food is your medicine".** I had to make the message as simple and as clear as possible and that's how I came up with **"Fresh is Best Forget the Rest"**. And this is my contribution.

FOOD MEDICINE: The Number#1 Rule to a Long and Healthy Life is just Volume 1. And more to follow. Look out for my next book "FOOD MEDICINE: THE REMEDY" and sign up on my website for more **'food medicine'**. www.happyhomesnz.com

Until then this is my offering to YOU with love.

REFERENCES

1/ https://books.google.co.nz/books?id=P7HGDQAAQBAJ&p-g=PT15&lpg=PT15&dq=US+studies+have+shown+pectin+al-so+protects+us+from+the+ravages+of+pollution,+binding+to+heavy+-metals+such+as+lead+or+mercury+in+the+body+and+carry-ing+them+safely+out.&source=bl&ots=MvxAZQjmB_&sig=AC-fU3U0RgW9CuYpgKxbWMdECvflwnrhNQg&hl=en&sa=X-&ved=2ahUKEwjqpdvi-MDmAhXRX3wKHX5wDRYQ6A-EwAHoECAQQAQ#v=onepage&q=US%20studies%20have%20shown%20pectin%20also%20protects%20us%20from%20the%20ravages%20of%20pollution%2C%20binding%20to%20heavy%20metals%20such%20as%20lead%20or%20mercury%20in%20the%20body%20and%20carrying%20them%20safely%20out.&f=false

2/ https://megustacoffee.com/specialty-coffee-online/benefits-to-using-apple-cider-vinegar-for-your-dogs-health/

3/ https://facty.com/lifestyle/wellness/what-is-pectin-what-does-it-do/4/

4/ https://onlinelibrary.wiley.com/doi/abs/10.1111/j.1365-2621.1976.tb14379.x

5/ https://www.medsafe.govt.nz/profs/datasheet/l/Loseccap.pdf

6/ https://ipfs.io/ipfs/QmXoypizjW3WknFiJnKLwHCnL72vedxj QkDDP1mXWo6uco/wiki/Four_thieves_vinegar.html

7/ https://www.ncbi.nlm.nih.gov/pubmed/4792931

8/ https://www.thejournal.ie/readme/vitamins-in-garlic-help-your-body-fight-carcinogens-and-get-rid-of-toxins-2623641-Feb2016/

9/ https://www.byrdie.com/sulfur-acne-treatments

10/ https://www.wcrf.org/dietandcancer

11/ https://www.consumeraffairs.com/news04/2005/pancreatic_cancer.html

12/ https://www.livescience.com/36057-truth-nitrites-lunch-meat-preservatives.html

13/ https://iskconnews.org/processed-meats-declared-too-dangerous-for-human-consumption,2887/

14/ https://www.indigo-herbs.co.uk/natural-health-guide/benefits/oat-grass

15/ https://www.greenmedinfo.health/disease/food-allergies

16/ https://www.healthyfoodguide.com.au/articles/2013/october/truth-about-carbs-weight-control

17/ https://www.nytimes.com/1982/05/03/business/advertising-bringing-stouffer-s-to-tv.html

18/ https://slideplayer.com/slide/5807301/

19/ http://www.stuff.co.nz/business/9828636/Consumers-shun-frozen-meals

20/ http://www.stuff.co.nz/business/9828636/Consumers-shun-frozen-meals

21/ https://en.wikipedia.org/wiki/Weston_Price

22/ https://mayooshin.com/blue-zones-diet/

23/ https://www.independent.co.uk/life-style/health-and-families/health-news/vitamin-pills-are-a-waste-of-money-offer-no-health-benefits-and-could-be-harmful-study-9010303.html

24/ https://www.newlight.com/

25/ https://www.dictionary.com/browse/paradichlorobenzene

26/ https://www.ecochem.co.nz/order-chemicals/uncategorised/chemico-paste/

27/ https://www.peacehealth.org/medical-topics/id/hn-2129002

28/ https://www.drroyallee.com/

29/ https://www.koanga.org.nz/shop/

30/ https://www.latimes.com/archives/la-xpm-2010-aug-08-la-ed-chemistry-20100808-story.html

31/ https://ourworldindata.org/life-expectancy

32/ http://naviauxlab.ucsd.edu/

33/ https://www.stitcher.com/podcast/india-kieser/the-doctors-farmacy-with-mark-hyman-md

34/ https://www.ncbi.nlm.nih.gov/pmc/articles/PMC5579676/

35/ https://experiencelife.com/article/8-hidden-toxins-whats-lurking-in-your-cleaning-products/

36/ https://www.dailymail.co.uk/health/article-185034/Can-deodo rants-cause-cancer.html

37/ https://www.healthpost.co.nz/body-crystal/?gclid=CjwKC AiA5o3vBRBUEiwA9PVzakeLxTfCGLQ9HQWWZpNeBU sbDb_1AvBU6pqIPahUhL2ELuvtCqVHmBoCFCEQAvD_ BwE&sort=bestselling

38/ https://www.nourishedlife.com.au/organic-shampoo/?job=10 36&action=click&channel_code=search&trfc=1&obj=3&utm_ source=GOOGLE&utm_medium=cpc&utm_campaign=NLOM-Dynamic-HairCare-Shampoo/Conditioner-AON&keyword=DY NAMIC+SEARCH+ADS&campaignid=71700000054226179& adgroupid=58700005147643808&kwid=p45294582032&tracke rid=39700045294582032&gclsrc=aw.ds&gclid=CjwKCAiA5o3vB RBUEiwA9PVzap6lBKdMiQTF60J4XXGcv3bpLRde7rOHBAx1 cbdARX7-XatlV_hKkRoCN9QQAvD_BwE&gclsrc=aw.ds

39/ https://naturvital.co.nz/category/hair-colour/?gclid=CjwKCAiA5o 3vBRBUEiwA9PVzaochJG1PtH1HKVFkhtNJc1_moKpnWXW16_ sZ-pMBasnIXRBMNbYtURoCK74QAvD_BwE